'I truly be [✓ KU-743-673] ...provides the reader with something that cannot be learned in medical textbooks... There is a wealth of real life experiences in this book to enable...the best possible care to people living with dementia.'

— *Tommy Dunne, living with dementia*

'This is essential reading for acute hospital healthcare professionals caring for people with dementia. Insightful case studies link evidence based frameworks to practical ways of improving care for people with dementia in hospital. Its accessible format means you can quickly dip into the issues relevant for you.'

— *Michelle Parker RN MSc BN (Hons), Lecturer in Adult Nursing, University of London*

'This book is both interesting and helpful in many different ways providing practical advice and possible solutions to help staff to consider the person and their psychological/social needs and not simply as the "confused" patient with a physical ailment. This book should be on every shelf of every ward!'

— *Caroline Baker, Director of Dementia Care at Barchester Healthcare and author of* Developing Excellent Care for People Living with Dementia in Care Homes

'This book is an excellent reminder of why patient-centred care is important and desirable for everyone concerned with the outcomes of hospital admission for people with dementia. It outlines logical ways of delivering care that are supported by evidence and also makes the argument for efficiency which is important in the current climate. Its simplicity is its strength.'

— *Vicki Leah, consultant nurse*

Excellent Dementia Care in Hospitals

A Guide to Supporting People with Dementia and their Carers

Jo James, Beth Cotton, Jules Knight, Rita Freyne, Josh Pettit and Lucy Gilby
With contributions by Nicci Gerrard and Julia Jones

Foreword by Tommy Dunne

Jessica Kingsley *Publishers*
London and Philadelphia

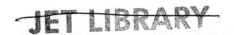

Photo on p.11 is reproduced with kind permission of Andy Paradise.

Triangle of care (Figure 2.2) is reproduced with kind permission of the Carers Trust.

First published in 2017
by Jessica Kingsley Publishers
73 Collier Street
London N1 9BE, UK
and
400 Market Street, Suite 400
Philadelphia, PA 19106, USA

www.jkp.com

Library of Congress Cataloging in Publication Data
A CIP catalog record for this book is available from the Library of Congress

British Library Cataloguing in Publication Data
A CIP catalogue record for this book is available from the British Library

ISBN 978 1 78592 108 7
eISBN 978 1 78450 372 7

Printed and bound in Great Britain

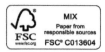

Contents

Royalties from this book will be donated to the Imperial Charity.

Foreword

Tommy Dunne

For too long there has been a need to equip healthcare professionals with the right knowledge and approach to be able to provide my peers (those living with dementia) and our carers with the very best possible care.

But how can you really provide care for someone if you don't fully understand the needs of those who require that care? After all, there are no manuals detailing case studies or the different scenarios that may occur.

You can't teach empathy, but you can teach people how to understand the needs of others and, from that, empathy can be born. Unfortunately, for too long there has been a care system in place of 'one size fits all'. At present there is nothing outside the norm to give guidance to health professionals about the different scenarios that they may face when dealing with people with dementia.

Behavioural problems in people with dementia are always triggered, and it's time to recognise that it is not just because a person has dementia. Health professionals need to get away from the age old belief that everything can be attributed to the dementia.

To truly deliver excellent care is about approach, understanding and caring enough to find out about the patient. I truly believe that this book provides the reader with something that cannot be learned from medical textbooks – it allows the reader to see and emotionally feel how a person with dementia experiences a stay in care, and it allows you to understand why a person with dementia who is admitted to hospital has a higher mortality rate, longer length of stay and is less likely to be discharged to their own home than other patients.

It's not surprising that those with dementia do not thrive in the hospital setting, which is intimidating for anyone, but for a person with dementia, it can be destabilising, lonely and terrifying. That's why this book recognises through John's Campaign that carers have a right to accompany their loved ones in hospital, and that carers can be in great need of a respite themselves.

There is a wealth of real life experiences in this book to enable those of you who really want to provide the best possible care to people living with dementia when they find themselves in hospital.

Tommy Dunne
Living with dementia

Introduction

This is Dianne Campbell. Dianne works at Imperial College Healthcare NHS Trust as a trainer and has lived with dementia for five years. If Dianne needs hospital care, like all of us, she wants to be treated like a person. She wants the staff to understand what matters to her 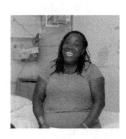 and she wants to be in control of her situation.

This book is not about protocols and policies and it is not about absolutes. It is about people. People who share similarities because of a diagnosis of dementia but have their own opinions, wishes, histories and hang-ups, just like everyone else.

As healthcare professionals, we need to change the approach from 'one size fits all' and 'it's because of the dementia' to something new. We must put the diagnosis of dementia to one side and find the person. When we have done that, we can start to make plans and decisions based on that person's needs and preferences, and we can start to understand what that person is trying to tell us and how best to support them in the bewildering hospital environment. This is what good dementia care looks like.

It can be done in the acute setting because delivering excellent care is about approach, understanding and caring enough to find out about the patient. Achieving this is within the reach of every healthcare professional. The aim of this book is to equip healthcare professionals in hospital settings with the right knowledge and approach to ensure that they can provide the best possible care to people living with dementia when they find themselves in hospital.

After exploring the role of carers and the theory under-pinning person-centred care, each chapter will use a case study to frame the narrative and to explore the evidence base in that area. In the 'How to make best practice happen' sections throughout the book, you will see a series of questions and answers relating to the subject matter and the case discussed earlier.

The chapters explore an issue that impacts on a person's well-being when in hospital. Sylvia and Sarah look at the complexities around discharge and decision making, exploring the role of the healthcare professional balanced against the rights and wishes of the person. Patrick focuses on communication and how to be effective in a busy clinical environment. Physical difficulties such as frailty, falls, vision, hearing, delirium, pain and eating and drinking are examined in John', Jaheem', Bridget' and Myrtle's chapters. How to get a person moving and engage them in meaningful activity is looked at in Geoffrey' and Miriam's chapters, and the impact of the hospital environment in Frank's chapter. Kenny's chapter considers what a healthcare professional can do on encountering different behaviour that can be hard to understand and gives the reader tips on how to approach patients exhibiting this in hospital. In Nicky and Denise's chapter, the end of life in dementia is addressed, with an emphasis on the impact of this on the carer. We finish with Stan's chapter, an exploration of the relevance and importance of touch when caring for a person with dementia in hospital.

This will show how enhanced understanding and knowing what questions to ask can restructure the approach to dementia care in hospital and redirect it towards a person-centred and strength-based model of care without using complicated planning tools.

ABOUT DEMENTIA

Before we start, it is perhaps important to clarify what we mean when we talk about dementia. When a group of people living with dementia was asked to choose the most accurate description of their illness, they choose this:

> Dementia is a syndrome that can be caused by over 100 different disorders in which there is deterioration in cognitive function (i.e. the ability to process thought) beyond what might be expected from normal ageing. It affects memory, thinking, orientation, comprehension, calculation, learning capacity, language, and judgment. (World Health Organisation 1990)

This means that damage to the brain changes the way a person thinks and acts. Another way of considering dementia is as causing a 'shift in the way a person experiences the world' (Power 2014). All dementias, regardless of the underlying disease, cause increasing physical frailty as they progress and life expectancy will be on average 7–12 years after diagnosis (Department of Health 2009).

Because people with dementia are often more frail and can be accident-prone, a large number of them will require hospital services. On average approximately 25 per cent of people in hospital will have dementia at any one time. In spite of the fact that this has been the case for many years, hospitals still struggle to meet the needs of people with dementia and subsequently they have worse outcomes than others. A person with dementia who is admitted to hospital has a higher mortality rate, longer length of stay and is less likely to be discharged to their own home (Dementia Action Alliance 2012).

Chapter 1

The Role and Importance of Carers in Hospital

Nicci Gerrard and Julia Jones

Hospitals are dangerous places for the old, the frail and those with delirium and dementia. It is increasingly accepted that they should not go there unless absolutely necessary and they should leave as soon as it is safe for them to do so. People with dementia often decline rapidly in hospital, both physically and mentally. This decline can create a vicious circle: they can't be discharged until they are better; they can't get better until they are discharged. Patients with dementia tend to stay longer than their peers without the condition; in their diminished condition, they are less likely to return to their own homes and they are more likely to be readmitted within 30 days (Alzheimer's Society 2009). It is common for them to become dehydrated, malnourished, incontinent and less mobile. Above all, they frequently become more confused and less independent. These are accepted facts – and they are also individual stories of distress and even tragedy. John's Campaign, which fights for the right of carers to accompany their loved ones in hospital and for the rights of those with dementia to be so accompanied, has collected numerous examples of catastrophic decline and unnecessary death (Gerrard and Jones 2016).

It's not surprising that those with dementia do not thrive in a hospital setting, which is intimidating for anyone and for them can be destabilising, lonely and terrifying. They need careful, kind, vigilant, person-centred care – to be treated not just as a patient with a particular condition that needs treating but as a vulnerable and precarious person. Good, compassionate nurses can do this: they can feed them and keep them mobile; they can listen to them. But they cannot know their history, understand their needs when they struggle painfully to articulate them and keep them connected to the world they have left behind when they enter hospital. A carer can be the voice for the patient who has no voice, their memory, their familiar face. They can be the patient's bridge to the professional world of nurses, doctors and therapists – the invaluable missing link.

Yet, in many hospitals in the UK, carers are not allowed to accompany people with dementia when they go into hospital. Kept out by rigid visiting hours, by rules that have grown up in a system that no longer exists and which now make little sense, everyone loses. The nurses lose part of the team of support around the patient, without whom their job becomes even harder and more stressful. The carer loses because they are prevented from being with the person they love at their time of need, and because they will have to suffer the physical and emotional consequences of a decline. Of course, the person with dementia loses – and what they lose can be everything, their whole self.

But lose-lose can be win-win. Where carers are welcomed, recognised as crucial and their expertise harnessed, then nurses are freer to nurse and the patient can be supported throughout their hospital stay. There is a growing body of evidence that involving carers reduces falls, malnutrition, dehydration and cognitive decline and also reduces the length of stay and the likelihood of swift readmission. On every level, it makes sense.

Although this is much harder to measure, involving the carer increases well-being and security and protects the patient's dignity and sense of self. It is a matter of compassion and decency that frail and vulnerable people who may be reaching the end of their life are accompanied. While John's Campaign (2016) has gathered numerous cases of the distress and decline of people with dementia while in hospital, it has also collected stories of terrific, compassionate practice, kindness in action – stories where staff went out of their way to welcome carers and make them feel recognised, and where patients were supported through their stay (Gerrard and Jones 2016).

John's Campaign argues that carers have a right to accompany their loved ones in hospital, but never a duty: carers can be in great need of a respite themselves. It understands that people with dementia often do not have carers. It knows that, for nursing staff, allowing carers into the world of the hospital is not a simple question of opening doors – they have to consider the privacy of other patients, the impact on staff time, the necessity of differentiating between visitors and carers and the importance of clearly communicating with the carer, so that everybody understands what their roles are and what their boundaries are. They might want to introduce carers' passports or lanyards, provide them with reclining chairs should they wish to stay overnight, offer them reduced parking charges or give them tea or even meal vouchers.

In hospitals in the UK that now have open access for carers, there are many examples of staff who have not simply allowed carers in but welcomed them with generosity, and who have enacted the principle of compassionate care with empathy and imagination. Up and down the country, hospital staff have gone beyond their job description to introduce dementia gardens, memory walks, murals on walls (and on ceilings of the theatre, for patients before their operation), music, shared mealtimes, therapeutic activities and events (Gerrard and Jones 2016). Such things, along with the presence of those people who mean the most to the person with dementia, give normal life the chance to flow into hospital spaces so that the safety of home doesn't feel so very far away.

From a carer's point of view, being welcomed into a mutually respectful working partnership can bring a form of respite that is not simple time-out. Too many carers are carrying a burden of anxiety and responsibility unsupported by professionals in the community. Not because social workers, district nurses, community mental health nurses, consultant psychiatrists, therapists, dementia specialist nurses are uncaring but they are so scarce, so overstretched. Being unable to access something as basic as timely continence advice and regular, appropriate supplies, for instance, can bring carers to breaking point (Newbronner *et al.* 2013). If there were better investment in community services, there would undoubtedly be fewer hospital admissions.

Carers may well be stressed and sleep-deprived – the period leading up to a hospital admission is likely to have been more than usually difficult – nevertheless a ban on their visits, a negation of all the time and thought they have already expended and an apparent disinterest in the fund of knowledge they have built up is not the way to offer respite. It is very much more likely to fuel suspicion, guilt and anger. If a family arrives all guns blazing, medical professionals should bear in mind that this may be the culmination of months of emotional and practical strain as well as the natural anxiety of a hospital admission. Many carers feel they are constantly running to catch up – and that their struggle is unwinnable. Potentially, there could be a measure of relief when a carer reaches a place where responsibility can be shared with a multidisciplinary team.

However, a concerned carer has invested so much of themselves in the person who depends on them that they are likely to be protective, defensive, unnecessarily thin-skinned. One of the strengths of the 2016–17 NHS England John's Campaign CQUIN (Commissioning for Quality and Innovation) is its insistence that hospital staff be trained in carer awareness (NHS England 2016). Some hospitals are already developing materials to facilitate this, working together with their local carer support organisations (for example, Newcastle Teaching Hospitals). One in three of all of us – hospital staff included – are likely to have caring responsibilities at some point in our lifetime, not just for people living with dementia but for people with learning difficulties, physical disabilities or a multitude of other life-limiting conditions, including our relatives' end-of-life period – for which we are often woefully unprepared and where there are no second chances. These responsibilities test our resilience and our humanity but they can also make us tricky to deal with. A nurse, doctor, therapist, hospital cleaner, volunteer who understands some of the pressures of informal caring can do so much to help validate carers to themselves and may then tap into a reservoir of expertise that is entirely essential to best patient care (Hannan *et al.* 2015).

On a pragmatic level, complaints reduce when carers are welcomed and satisfaction levels increase. Communication is improved and this aspect alone is an immeasurable benefit to the chances of successful treatment. Initially, doctors or therapists may grumble about the extra time spent explaining their courses of action to carers as well as to the patient but this is an investment in that person's future. Who is going to check that newly prescribed medication continues to be taken correctly after the patient leaves hospital? Who will be encouraging and supervising suggested exercises? Overloading families (or care home staff) with a welter of important information on discharge day is very much less efficient than spending a little extra time including them in the multidisciplinary team discussions during the in-patient stay. Likewise, offering direct support for the family carer themselves is an additional precaution against early readmission. There are plenty of carer organisations ready to work with hospitals on this and a word at the right moment from a member of the hospital staff will go a long way to ensuring that any available external support is at least considered.

Before the critical moment of a hospital admission, carers may not know that they are carers – they may not fully realise how much their day-to-day support matters to the well-being of the person living with dementia. Similarly, the patient may not be aware of the extent of their dependence until after it has been denied them, by which time there will be the beginning of avoidable harm. Hospitals whose procedures prompt the involvement of carers (whether family, friends or paid help) from admission until discharge are serving their patients well.

The extent of involvement during the stay will naturally vary with the carer's availability and other commitments – just because someone is supporting her elderly father doesn't necessarily mean she hasn't also got children to take to school or a job to hold down. Carers are often suffering financially as a direct result of the time they are already giving. Hospital policies that enable a carer to continue support at the times that suit her or his other responsibilities – rather than demanding they be corralled into hospital visiting hours – not only assist sustainability but may also help keep the patient better orientated.

A hospital admission is hugely disruptive – though obviously necessary in the good cause of healing. Someone living with dementia may not seem clear whether it is day or night or may feel lost even within their own homes but they may also be more alert to small clues than they are able to express. If a mother is used to her son popping in every morning on his way to work and he is encouraged to continue while she is in hospital, his visit at that accustomed time may offer an almost imperceptible anchor to normality. A nurse who takes the trouble to learn from the regular giver both when and how a patient is used to receiving medication has more chance of seeing it accepted. In the case of patients who are living with Parkinson's (where precise timing is crucial) such small person-centred adjustments take on a whole new level of clinical importance (Parkinson's UK 2016). In other cases it will be the hospital admission itself that brings unexpected new responsibilities for carers or prompts a radical reappraisal of their current situation. In these cases too, working together during the in-patient stay should make the subsequent transition easier.

Hospitals which are considering offering a 24/7 welcome to carers may feel panicked by the prospect of numbers of people crowding the wards or by the particular difficulties of overnight stays. They need not be. No carer is going to want to stay overnight unless they are convinced that the person they care for really needs their presence – usually to ward off the dangers of extreme confusion, fear and, potentially, delirium. In this case it is clearly in the hospital's best interests (and the interests of its other patients) to make whatever arrangements are necessary to facilitate the stay. Then, after a night or two, if all goes well, trust will have been established, the patient settled and the carer will be glad of a chance to sleep at home 'on call'.

Staff anxieties that welcoming carers onto the wards will cause overcrowding, bring disturbance to other patients, make it more difficult to maintain cleanliness or to undertake certain more delicate or invasive procedures should not be ignored but should be addressed (Charalambous 2016). Numbers per patient can be managed with a passport system or a carer's card. Anti-infection procedures can be explained on admission – carers are the last people to want to see the person they look after picking up some hospital superbug. It is simply nonsense for cleaners to say, for instance, that they couldn't clean properly around a bed because there was someone sitting next to it. Explain the need and the carer will move, pick up their chair and probably offer to shift the locker as well. A ward full of educated carers is potentially a ward full of vigilant hygiene hawks. All the problems of co-existing in a patient-focused community can be addressed in the same way: through education, explanation and empathy. Encourage carers to reflect how they would want their own relative's privacy respected and there is unlikely to be any resistance if they are asked to leave the bay for a short time while the person in the next bed is receiving personal care. Clearly written information leaflets are invaluable in setting out mutual expectations, codes of conduct and responsibilities. An attitude of teamwork and willing patient-focused partnership, established from day one, is better still.

Carers are not a magic bullet for the NHS and its most vulnerable patients. For a start, the figures do not add up. There are 800,000 people living with dementia and 670,000 carers. One in five adults is ageing without children and others may be separated by distance or permanently estranged. There is a heart-stopping rise in the number of people over 85 who are carers themselves either for their partners or for ageing disabled children (Newbronner *et al.* 2013). Caring is a relationship-based activity that tests relationships to their limits. There will be days when even the most sensitive and devoted carer cannot assuage the distress of the person they love – and who loves them. Some people with dementia may be emotionally manipulative or bullying. Some carers can be angry or abusive.

It's as well to be honest about these issues because, however difficult it may be to establish caring partnerships, nothing will make the plight of people with dementia in hospital go away. If there is a willing carer able to act as the 'cognitive ramp' for any single one of these patients, for any period of their stay, hospitals should fling their arms wide to embrace them.

Nicci Gerrard and **Julia Jones** are authors and founders of John's Campaign, which advocates for the right to stay with people with dementia in the hospital.

Chapter 2

Principles Underpinning Good Care

Until recently, the care of people with dementia has been dominated by a discourse around deficits and the care plan is likely to be concentrated on what the patient is unable to do and how this will impact on their lives and abilities. While, in many situations, this is a pragmatic approach to care, it is also a negative one and one that sets up an expectation of failure and loss from the onset.

When we change the dialogue to one around enablement and disablement, and think of a person who is being disabled by a combination of factors that includes cognitive and functional deficits but also encompasses social, societal and emotional factors, we can start to view the care of people with dementia in a different way. 'The focus on disease and deficits has held us back in understanding' (Feil 2002, p.65).

DISABLING BEHAVIOUR

In 1997, Kitwood's work *Dementia Reconsidered* identified the ways in which a person with dementia can be disabled by the behaviour of others and named this 'malignant social psychology'. In Table 2.1 we can see how malignant social psychology is present in acute care, often unconsciously applied by staff who might be unaware of the effect it can have on the patient.

Table 2.1: The presence of malignant social psychology in hospitals

Item	What it means	What we do in hospitals
Treachery	Deception to distract or manipulate a person or make them comply.	'Your son will be back in a minute' (when you know he is not coming). 'If you do this, we'll let you go home.'
Disempowerment	Not allowing the person to use the abilities they do have – not helping them to complete tasks they have started.	Feeding and washing patients when they can feed or wash themselves with help because it is quicker.
Infantilisation	Patronising a person.	Calling an older person 'sweetie' and 'love'. Comments like 'She's so sweet'.
Intimidation	Inducing fear in a person, through the use of threats or physical power.	Using implied threats. 'If you don't agree to this you will get worse/we won't be able to help you anymore.'
Labelling	Using a category such as dementia as the main basis for interacting with a patient and explaining their behaviour.	'She always does that – it's her dementia.'
Stigmatisation	Treating the person as if they are a diseased object or an outcast.	'It's upsetting for the other patients, they should have a special ward for them.'
Outpacing	Providing information, presenting choices at a rate too fast for a person to understand, putting them under pressure to do things more rapidly than they can bear.	'You need to have surgery for an obstruction in your bowel, we need to take some blood and consent you before the operation, any questions?'

Invalidation	Failing to acknowledge the subjective reality of a person's experience, especially what they are feeling.	'She's not really upset, she's completely doolally – thinks she's at home.'
Objectification	Treating the person as if they were a lump of dead matter; to be pushed, lifted, filled, pumped or drained without proper reference to the fact they are sentient beings.	'Roll him over. Pass me the cloth, I'll wash his back. There, can you do the front? Let's sit him up to eat after this.'
Ignoring	Carrying on (conversation or action) in the presence of a person as if they were not there.	Staff talking to each other while delivering care. 'How was your weekend?'
Imposition	Forcing a person to do something, overriding desire or denying the possibility of choice on their part.	'I'm afraid there's no option, you have to do this.'
Withholding	Refusing to give attention or to meet a need.	Ignoring a patient who is calling out because the person has dementia.
Accusation	Blaming a person for actions or failures arising from their lack of ability or misunderstanding.	'Why did you do that?' 'That's disgusting.'
Disruption	Intruding suddenly on a person's action or reflection; crudely breaking their frame of reference.	Interrupting a patient who is trying to tell you something when you are in a hurry.
Mockery	Making fun of a person's 'strange' actions, teasing, humiliating, and making jokes at their expense.	'She's hilarious, come and see what she does when you try and get her to walk.'
Disparagement	Telling a person they are incompetent, useless and worthless, giving them messages that are damaging to their self-esteem.	'No you can't do that.' 'You are not strong enough to lift that anymore.'

Before we explore how staff can enable people with dementia and enhance well-being, we need to ensure that we are not creating the problem by the kind of behaviours and attitudes that are shown in Table 2.1.

WHY WELL-BEING?

When trying to describe a desired state for a person with dementia, theorists have often struggled to find a term to encompass a sense of *being in a good place* or the combination of factors which make a person feel right. The term 'well-being' is increasingly used to describe a state which can exist in spite of physical illness and disability and has a major impact on the lives of people with dementia.

The World Health Organisation (1948) defined health as 'a state of optimal well-being, not merely the absence of disease and infirmity', illustrating how important well-being is in the context of healthcare. The dimensions of well-being are described as a balance of physical, mental, emotional, environmental, spiritual and social factors.

For people with dementia, the discourse on well-being has evolved from the realities of hostile and dehumanising care environments with malignant social psychology. These environments have given rise to the concept of ill-being in dementia, and evidence has shown that many of the common problems cited in dementia care such as behavioural problems and refusal arise from the person's state of ill-being.

Kitwood suggested that well-being in dementia can be achieved through a combination of interlinked factors which meet human needs such as identity, inclusion and security. A representation of this model, based on Kitwood's flower (Kitwood 1997), is shown in Figure 2.1. For individuals with dementia, these simple foundations of personhood and contentment will be harder to achieve particularly as the disease progresses.

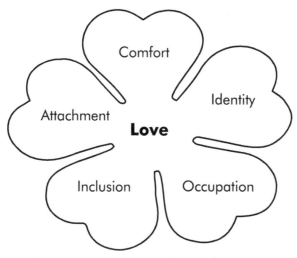

Figure 2.1: A representation of Kitwood's principles

It is important to note that the foundation of well-being in Kitwood's model does not rely on physical health and can therefore be applied in the hospital setting when a person is unwell. The challenge for staff working in the busy hospital environment is to find a way to ensure that the patient's well-being is considered as a valuable part of the therapeutic approach and that it does not lose out to clinical processes and rigid routines.

STRENGTH-BASED CARE

By combining a strength-based and person-centred approach to care, the staff member can ensure that the person with dementia receives care which meets the essential need for well-being as well as meeting the person's physical needs.

In 2004, the EDGE Programme (Ronch *et al.* 2004) used the concept of strength-based care planning for people with dementia, changing the focus from something perceived as a problem to finding the strength associated with that activity (see Table 2.2).

**Table 2.2: An example of strength-based
care planning using the EDGE Model**

Domain	Problem/Strength	Goal/Approach
Biological	*Problem:* Weight loss.	*Goal:* Gerald will gain 1lb in the next month.
	Strength: Is able to eat certain finger foods with limited assistance. Gerald is able to drink.	*Approach:* 1) Provide finger foods that Gerald will be able to eat without difficulty. 2) Staff to sit with Gerald at mealtimes to assist him if necessary.
Activities of daily living	*Problem:* Unsafe wandering.	*Goal:* Gerald will walk around the building regularly without falling or exiting when provided with verbal cues.
	Strength: Able to walk independently. Likes to walk when there is something to do or see.	*Approach:* 1) Staff will provide verbal cues when Gerald is mobilising. 2) Staff or family member will walk with Gerald to the coffee shop daily.

By using a strengths-based approach, we can truly break free of the limitations of a narrow biomedical view and realise successes that have been unattainable with our traditional approaches. Regardless of any future advances in medical therapy, well-being remains essential, and will never come out of a pill bottle. (Power 2015)

PERSON-CENTRED CARE

Kitwood, as cited by Dr Epp in his article 'Person-centred dementia care: a vision to be refined' (2003, p.15), strongly emphasised that 'person-centred care is founded on the ethic that all human beings are of absolute value and worthy of respect, no matter their disability, and on a conviction that people with dementia can live fulfilling lives'.

Person-centred care is perhaps one of the most pressing international discussions in present healthcare systems. It is a way of thinking and doing things that sees individuals using health and social services as equal partners in planning, developing and monitoring care to ensure it meets their care needs. This means putting people and their families at the heart of decisions and viewing them as experts, working alongside professionals to get the best result.

Hospital staff are gradually moving away from a medical model of care towards one that is focused on the individual's care needs. As the concept of person-centred care gains more attention, it is vital that we make sure we understand what the term encompasses. Building a rapport with your patients can be difficult in the acute hospital setting with a fast turnover of patients, limited information and too much focus on time-based targets. Here, we will explore how hospital staff can find ways of achieving person-centred care in a hospital setting.

WHAT DOES PERSON-CENTRED CARE REALLY STAND FOR, AND WHY DO WE NEED IT TODAY?

There is promising evidence that many aspects of person-centred care are improving people's lives and making healthcare delivery more efficient. Based on this evidence, international policy now recommends that acute care for people with dementia should be informed by the principles of person-centred care and that interventions should be designed to sustain their individuality.

A core principle of person-centred care is that services should be moulded around each individual, as opposed to an individual being moulded around a service. As the old saying goes, 'Square pegs in round holes don't fit, no matter how hard you try to make them!'

There are four key principles of person-centred care and the success of each stage is dependent on the thoroughness and analysis of the information gathered:

- *Principle 1:* Being person-centred means affording people dignity, respect and compassion.

- *Principle 2:* Being person-centred means offering coordinated care, support or treatment.

- *Principle 3:* Being person-centred means offering personalised care, support or treatment.

- *Principle 4:* Being person-centred means being enabled.

In order to ensure a deep foundation of the principles of person-centred care, there must be a shared understanding of the role and mutual respect of the person with dementia, the staff member and the carer which all fit into the triangle of care (see Figure 2.2).

TRIANGLE OF CARE

The triangle of care describes the relationship between the person with dementia, the staff member and the carer, which promotes safety, supports communication and ultimately sustains well-being (Hannan *et al.* 2015). Person-centred care needs to be a partnership which recognises the relationship between the patient and the staff member, and therefore the significance of confidence and understanding. To achieve this partnership there must be recognition that optimal health outcomes can only be attained by collaboration and the sharing of knowledge and expertise within a restorative relationship, and an alliance within the triangle of care. The National Institute for Health and Care Excellence (NICE) and the Social Care Institute for Excellence (SCIE) (2006) emphasise the importance of relationships and interactions with others to the individual with dementia, and their potential for promoting well-being in the delivery of person-centred care.

The Health Innovation Network (2016) acknowledged that the following aspects/factors are required to deliver person-centred care:

- Respecting an individual's values and putting them at the centre of care.

- Taking into account an individual's preferences and enabling them to express their needs; ensuring that their care is coordinated and integrated.

- Working together to ensure that there is good communication and information.

- Ensuring that patients are physically comfortable and safe.

- Providing emotional support; involving family and carers; making sure that there is continuity between and within services.

- Making sure that people have access to appropriate care as and when they need it.

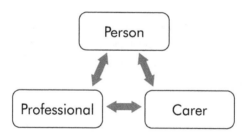

Figure 2.2: The triangle of care (Hannan *et al.* 2015)

WHAT ARE THE BENEFITS OF PERSON-CENTRED CARE?

Research has found that person-centred care has made a big impact on the quality of care. Tritter and Koivusalo (2013) highlighted the following outcomes:

- *Improved quality of life* for those with dementia can be acquired when people are involved in social activities and encouraged to become engaged in their past pleasures.

Person-centred care can also help in sustaining a symbiotic relationship between the carer and the person affected by dementia, which in turn can maintain the care recipient's high level of psychological well-being and productive behaviours, hence reducing depression.

- *Better sleep patterns.* Respecting past interests and current capabilities can improve sleep during the night and daytime napping, as shown in person-centred care research programmes.

- *Less agitation.* Studies have shown that decreased agitation can be achieved in person-centred care programmes if we respect the client's freedom of choice regarding the individual's daily routine. This can lead to decreased verbal agitation and also ward staff feeling less rushed and more tolerant to clients' behaviours.

- *Improved self-esteem.* Research indicates that when people with dementia are being provided with the opportunity of expressing themselves and their needs, they will maintain a positive sense of self. This can significantly reduce their feelings of grief, anxiety, anger and feeling like a burden to others.

- People are being encouraged to lead a more *healthy lifestyle,* such as exercising or eating healthily.

- More *collaborative decision making* about individuals care needs, which ensures appropriate onward referrals being made.

- Probable reduction in the overuse of services, which in turn will have a reduction in the overall *cost of care.*

- Increased levels of *staff satisfaction* and confidence about the care provided.

HOW DO WE INITIATE PERSON-CENTRED CARE?

Here are five strategies to support person-centred care based on a care-assessment tool research study:

1. Gather relevant information about the person's past, likes and dislikes, and incorporate these into the care giving.

2. Ensure that no task or aspect of care is placed higher than the subjective experience of the individual.

3. Make all routines and activities flexible for the person with dementia, so that they can be easily adapted according to individual's wishes.

4. Facilitate reminiscence with appropriate stimuli.

5. Take into consideration and acknowledge the importance of the individual's own interpretation of their subjective reality.

GATHERING RELEVANT INFORMATION

It is paramount to ensure that the patient can maintain their identity; therefore staff must get to see who the patient is that they are providing care to. Patients want staff to know what is important to them, and relatives want staff to value what they know about the patient.

BEING VERSUS DOING

Being person-centred means that when we plan care with the person, we think about the effect of what we're doing on the person as a whole. For example, when a young female healthcare support worker (HCSW) plans to assist an elderly man with bathing, the stages of the activity are very straightforward – ensure that the water temperature and depth are appropriate, that any adapted equipment is working and is used properly and that the person's dignity is protected, and complete the task with the man feeling clean and refreshed. The HCSW is perfectly competent to ensure that all these components are addressed.

But what might the older man feel about being bathed by a young woman who might be no older than his own daughter, or even granddaughter? Will it make him feel helpless, humiliated or useless? Does he want a bath in the first place? When we begin to think of the care we give in this way – of the effect of what we're doing on the whole person – we're giving care in a person-centred way. That might mean compromise – the HCSW might, for instance, negotiate with the man and agree that for today a wash from a basin at the bedside or the bathroom will be sufficient.

There is a considerable amount we can do to promote an individual's safety. For example, ensuring that people are comfortable, that they call for us to be aware of the things that can cause discomfort – feeling cold or hot, having a thirst or being hungry, being in pain or having an itch, needing to go to the toilet or change a sitting position, for instance – and to take steps to relieve them. Having people's well-being uppermost means that nothing we do – or don't do – causes the individual any physical, emotional or social harm.

OPENING THE DOOR

It is important to attempt to place oneself in the shoes of the individual with dementia. In a busy, stressful, demanding and often chaotic hospital ward, this is not always easy. Nevertheless, seeing the world through the eyes of the person with dementia, if even for five minutes, can prove enlightening, time-saving and even life-saving.

The introduction of person-centred approaches to dementia care can have a positive impact on the interaction between the individual and ward staff, offering an opportunity for continuity of care, improved communication and preservation of the dignity of the person with dementia. This in turn can help alleviate some of the symptoms and responses of the person with dementia that hospital staff find difficult.

Although the treatment given helps with recovery from the illness, nurses who have been patients often report that it is the small things that matter. These include staff taking the time to stop and talk, and giving information and reassurance.

KNOWING THE PERSON: 'MY STORY'

Life story work is an activity which involves reviewing a person's past life events and developing a biography. It can be used in a care setting to support staff in understanding more about the individual and their experiences. It enhances the care provided to individuals with dementia. The benefits of life story work as an intervention for people with dementia and their families has been recognised for some time with regard to promoting person-centred care, improving assessment outcomes, building relationships between ward staff and family/carers as well as improving communication within the triangle of care (Thompson 2011). This is a person-centred thinking tool that can support people living with dementia in the transition from being passive recipients of care to them being recognised as vital members in this triangle of care.

Chapter 3

Sylvia – The Importance of Community Support and Discharge

Sylvia slipped on an icy pavement and was taken to the emergency department as she was unable to get up. Sylvia had fractured her right femur and had a hip replacement. Post-operatively, it has been noted that she has a hypoactive delirium and is being treated for a urinary tract infection (UTI). Her oral intake has declined significantly and she is described as 'non-engaging' and 'low in mood' in the medical notes.

She was diagnosed with Alzheimer's disease two years ago and lives with her dog, Champ, in a terraced cottage without any formal support. She originates from Jamaica and has lived in England most of her life with her husband and daughter, Grace. She worked as a domestic in her local hospital until she retired. She often talks about her late husband and Grace, who lives 300 miles away. Ted, her neighbour, occasionally gets her shopping or looks after Champ.

WHAT NEEDS TO BE IN PLACE FOR DISCHARGE?

When a person with dementia is admitted to hospital, discharge planning should start as soon as possible. In the case of an elective admission, this should start at the pre-assessment clinic and in emergency admissions within 24 hours of arrival. The patient's family should be involved where this is appropriate, as it is likely that they will provide invaluable information regarding the home situation and they can also provide a strong support network. However, it must be recognised that there may not be a family carer or they may not always be able to provide support on discharge.

The process of discharge planning relies on the outcome of the multidisciplinary team's assessments, and the plan should be developed in discussion with the patient and their main family carer. If the assessment determines that the patient needs little or no care, this is referred to as a *minimal discharge*, but if there are more complex needs and the patient requires specialised care, then this is referred to as a *complex discharge*.

Every hospital will have a local discharge policy, but many aspects of discharge planning are universal and staff need to understand the underlying principles of safe discharge. Clinicians on the ward are vital to the discharge process and need to be working on it throughout the patient's admission. Table 3.1 shows what needs to be done in the complex discharge process in the UK and what happens when it is not done.

Sylvia's recovery was hampered by the fluctuation in her cognitive state, with the team initially describing her as being 'way off her previous baseline and not engaging with therapies'. It was felt that her needs were complex for this reason.

Initially, it was thought that Sylvia may need to go into a care home, as she had deteriorated functionally and needed extensive support with regard to her care needs. It became evident, however, that Sylvia had delirium and when this was treated she began to improve and engage with staff. Plans for her discharge then changed focus towards her returning home with the support of a care package. Once Sylvia's delirium started to resolve she was able to make informed decisions about her care needs and plans for discharge. Some patients with dementia may not have capacity to make decisions about their future care needs and decisions will need to be made in their best interests (see Chapter 4).

Table 3.1: The discharge process

Time	What needs to be done	Why it needs to be done	Who can do it	Consequences of not doing it
24 hours	If there is a care need, a Section 2 form should be completed	This form tells social services that the person is in hospital and either needs a care package cancelling or alerts them to the potential need for a new care package.	Ward staff	Existing care package will not be cancelled. The patient might be charged for care while in hospital. This will cause a delay as social services will not pick up the patient straightaway.
Within two days of receipt of section 2	Social services assessment	The social worker will assess the patient's needs.	Social worker	No package of care can be organised or put into place until the patient has had a social services assessment.
Within one week	Multidisciplinary team (MDT) assessment of the patient	The MDT will discuss the patient's needs from a nursing, medical and therapies perspective and assess the level of care they will require.	MDT	Without this assessment, there will be no guidance as to what level of support the patient might need at home.
24 hours before discharge	Section 5 form	This form alerts social services to the imminent discharge so that they can get everything in place.	Ward teams	If social services do not receive this form, they will not start the package of care and the patient might go home and find that there is no support. This can lead to readmission to hospital.

WHAT HAPPENS WHEN A PERSON WITH DEMENTIA GOES HOME?

When a person with dementia initially returns home from hospital, even if they have recovered well and returned to their previous baseline of functioning, it is likely that there will be a period of adjustment, and a package of care will be need to support the transition.

The different terms for health and social care are often used interchangeably, in spite of the fact that they have clear differences. It is important for hospital clinicians to have a good understanding of what is available and how each service differs from the other. Often, it is nursing staff caring most closely for a patient like Sylvia who will be able to identify the best option for a patient when they are discharged.

In particular, there is confusion around the difference between intermediate care and reablement; services in different areas will vary depending on the interpretation of the terms. Therefore, it is important for the hospital clinician to identify and understand what each of the services in their own area offer.

INTERMEDIATE CARE

Age UK describes intermediate care as 'short-term NHS and/or social care support that aims to help you live independently at home for as long as possible' (Age UK 2016). Services that form part of intermediate care must be free for the first six weeks. If a local authority provides the services, they have the discretion to extend the free provision beyond six weeks. Intermediate care services is used as an umbrella term to describe the following:

- *Crisis response* – offering short-term care (usually 48–72 hours) and direct access to a dedicated team who can put support services into place at short notice. This is often implemented to avoid hospital admissions.

- *Reablement* – this is about helping people to regain or retain self-care function for themselves, rather than providing input that replaces it – for example, supporting someone to cook rather than providing meals on wheels (Parker 2014). On average, reablement packages last for six weeks after first visit. They are often used after hospital admissions – for example, after a person has had falls and lost confidence.

- *Enablement* – this provides someone with adequate power, means, opportunity or authority to do something (HarperCollins 1992). Enablement will often be used when a person has met their functional goals in hospital and needs long-term care.

Other forms of post-hospital care are rehabilitation and recovery, both of which have a place in supporting people with dementia:

- *Rehabilitation* – a process aimed at restoring personal autonomy in those aspects of daily living considered most relevant by the patients or service users and their family carers (Sinclair and Dickinson 1998). It is of upmost importance to remember that people with dementia do have the cognitive reserves required to engage in rehabilitation and they should always be considered as candidates for rehabilitation. The key to ensuring that people with dementia are considered for rehabilitation is through clear goal setting, which can prove the patient's rehabilitation potential.

- *Recovery* – this is about building a meaningful and satisfying life as defined by the person themselves, whether or not there are ongoing or recurring symptoms or problems. Recovery represents a move away from pathology, illness and symptoms to health, strength and wellness (Shepherd, Boardman and Slade 2008).

Initially, Sylvia was offered a short stay in a rehabilitation unit, but declined this as she wanted to go home. An extensive care package was then offered to Sylvia, but she felt that with the support of her daughter they could manage with her personal hygiene and meals. It was suggested that they begin with the full care package and reduce it accordingly, and they both agreed to this. After these negotiations, she was discharged home with a reablement package of care.

A micro-environment was set up in her lounge. This is usually a short-term solution for someone with reduced mobility. It involves setting up everything the person needs in one room or on one level. In Sylvia's case, this was a bed, a commode and an armchair. She had visits from a community physiotherapist and a community occupational therapist who recommended adaptations to her house which were made over the next few weeks, including grab rails by the front door and a second banister rail up the stairs so that she had extra support when mobilising up to her bedroom. This enabled Sylvia to return to her previous level of functioning and she no longer needed the micro-environment.

The financial impact of care is often a source of anxiety for people with dementia and their families. The clinician should ensure that the patient and family have access to a social worker so that they can discuss what is available to them and how to manage their finances going forward.

ONGOING SUPPORT IN THE COMMUNITY

Statutory services are central to ensuring a smooth discharge, and they can continue to support the person with dementia and the main carer in the community. However, there are also many third-sector services that can offer support, on a national and also local level, though the type and amount will be different in each area. The organisations detailed below have both national and local services, and an internet search will reveal what is available in local areas:

- Alzheimer's Society

- Age UK

- Dementia UK (Admiral Nurses and the Admiral Nursing Direct helpline)

- Carers Trust.

A ward must endeavour to build relationships with local organisations so that up-to-date information is available on the ward. It can be helpful to have local information on the ward, perhaps a noticeboard or a leaflet rack, as patients and relatives may not be aware of all the services they can access, such as memory cafes or befriending services. After discharge, Sylvia met with her local dementia adviser and she started attending the local dementia cafe on a weekly basis, and a befriender was organised for her through a local organisation which helped to reduce her sense of isolation. Grace also made contact with a local carers support group, and she has used the Admiral Nursing Direct helpline when she needed emotional support and practical advice in caring for her mother.

How to make best practice happen

Have I asked why Sylvia is reacting this way?	Sylvia is afraid that she will not be able to return home.
	When her neighbour, and later her daughter, arrived, staff had a clearer picture of Sylvia and understood her independence and desire to go home.
	Healthcare support workers will not usually be actively involved in discharge planning but can be helpful in gaining information from the patient and relaying to the appropriate teams.
What are Sylvia's strengths/ abilities?	Sylvia was able to express her needs and rights from the beginning of her admission.
	She had been looking after her dog Champ and her ability to do this was one of her strengths.
	These things show Sylvia was managing well at home prior to admission and that she has support.

	Qualified staff	Healthcare support worker
Am I listening?	Sylvia has expressed clearly that she wants to go home. Once her delirium resolved she has been able to take an active role in her discharge planning.	Sylvia expressed her wish to go home as soon as possible when she was admitted. Relay this information to the appropriate teams so Sylvia's preferred place for discharge is taken into account.
Do I know enough about Sylvia?	Get to know your patient's life story. Sylvia was a very sociable lady, but she had become isolated.	Talk to the patient. Ask her about her home and how long she has lived there. Discuss events and things that have happened while Sylvia has lived there. Relay any information to appropriate teams.
What can I do to enable Sylvia?	Listen to what Sylvia feels she needs and wants when she goes home. Use her ability to express herself to support planning. Make sure that Sylvia is facilitated to continue looking after Champ after discharge as this keeps her focused and helps her remain independent.	Ensure that you stay up to date with discharge plans for the patient. If you learn anything from Sylvia or her family and friends, be sure to inform the appropriate teams so this can be taken into account during the planning of her discharge and, it is hoped, help to get Sylvia back to her own home.

Chapter 4

Sarah – Making Decisions

Sarah is 78 years old and was diagnosed with vascular dementia five years ago. She was admitted to hospital with facial injuries after a fight with her partner. She does not want treatment and wants to return home. However, due to the seriousness of her injuries a safeguarding alert has been raised and she is not allowed to leave. Her partner has been arrested for assault. They have a close circle of friends who describe them as having a volatile relationship which often results in violence. Both Sarah and her partner have been admitted to hospital with injuries in the past. They have been together for 30 years and their friends describe them as inseparable. Sarah is extremely angry with staff and repeatedly tries to leave the ward to go home. She tells staff that they have 'no right' to keep her here.

Making decisions in healthcare can be complex and requires consideration of numerous different factors. Clinicians must act legally, ethically and professionally while ensuring that the best possible outcome is achieved for the patient. On the surface, it appears quite simple:

> Sarah needs to be treated and therefore we will treat her because we know that is the best thing for her – even if that means holding her down to do it.

This paternalistic approach to Sarah's care is common in healthcare settings; however, it fails to consider several factors that need to be addressed:

- Sarah has rights.

- We must act ethically.

- We must act legally.

- We might not know what is best for Sarah.

In 2015, the World Health Organisation released a thematic briefing on Human Rights for People Living with Dementia and stated that 'people living with Dementia should be empowered to participate in decision making processes' (World Health Organisation 2015).

SARAH'S RIGHTS

When we look at decision making for a person like Sarah, we must first consider her rights. Every person has human rights, which are fundamental. In 2000, the Human Rights Act came into force in the UK and made the principles outlined in the European Convention on Human Rights into British law. This means that when treating Sarah the clinical staff need to understand their actions in light of the 16 articles of the Human Rights Act as every public sector organisation must operate within the confines of the Act.

The articles which are relevant to healthcare professionals are:

- Article 2: The right to life.

- Article 3: The right not to be tortured or subjected to treatment which is inhumane or degrading.

- Article 5: The right to liberty and security.

It is particularly important to be aware of Sarah's rights and, as a clinician, to act as an advocate for her, because people with dementia are at high risk of having their human rights ignored, particularly when it comes to healthcare delivery.

ACTING ETHICALLY

All clinicians are aware of the need to act ethically; it is intrinsic to the various codes of practice which regulate their work. However, there is often confusion about the application of ethics to everyday care. In fact, ethics can be seen as exploring the question of the right thing to do and are relevant to all aspects of life. However, in situations where clinicians are required to make decisions which affect another person, the need to approach these decisions using an ethical framework is paramount.

Beauchamp and Childress's (2009) four essential components of ethical care (Autonomy, Beneficence, Non-Maleficence and Justice) clarify the responsibilities for the clinician and we can see how closely they sit with the articles of the Human Rights Act. However, when we consider this in light of Sarah's situation, we can also see that there is a moral tension as shown in Figure 4.1 below:

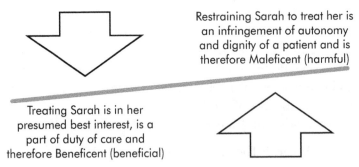

Restraining Sarah to treat her is an infringement of autonomy and dignity of a patient and is therefore Maleficent (harmful)

Treating Sarah is in her presumed best interest, is a part of duty of care and therefore Beneficent (beneficial)

Figure 4.1: The moral tension in Sarah's situation

Decision making in these situations is often a balancing act requiring the clinician to weigh up advantages and disadvantages and choose the best available option, even if there are still problems with that option. Moral tensions such as the one above commonly occur in healthcare settings and illustrate the importance of having a robust understanding of the structures and laws that are in place to protect both patients and staff from the misuse of position and power. The Mental Capacity Act can be used to support decision making not just for patients but also for staff who need guidance. Using the Act in relation to Sarah will be explored later in this chapter.

If a decision that has been made feels wrong, it is often because it *is* wrong, or at the very least has complexities that might need unpicking. In a sense, the cornerstone of ethical behaviour is not walking away from a situation that feels uncomfortable, but instead confronting it and acting as an advocate for the person in your care regardless of how difficult that might be.

MENTAL CAPACITY ACT

The Mental Capacity Act (2005) came into force in England and Wales in April 2007 and has changed the way in which decisions are made for adults who are deemed to lack capacity. The Act provides a legal framework for making decisions and acting on behalf of individuals who lack the mental capacity to make their own decisions.

The purpose of the Act is to support people in making decisions, and to ensure any decision or action taken on behalf of someone who lacks capacity is made in their best interests. These can be to do with day-to-day matters (such as what to wear, what to buy during weekly shopping) or major, potentially life-changing decisions.

The Act is underpinned by five principles:

- A person must be assumed to have capacity unless it is established that they lack it.

- A person is not to be treated as unable to make a decision unless all practical steps to help them to do so have been taken without success.

- A person is not to be treated as unable to make a decision simply because they make an unwise decision.

- An act done or decision made, under this Act, for or on behalf of a person who lacks capacity must be done, or made, in the person's best interests. Before the act is done, or the decision made, consideration must be given as to whether it is the least restrictive option.

In Sarah's case, a decision needs to be made regarding her receiving treatment. The team needs to assess her capacity in relation to this. Before assessing her capacity, there are things to consider. Is Sarah being fully supported to understand what is being discussed?

- If the patient does not speak English, ensure that there is a neutral (non-family) interpreter who will translate word for word what the patient says.

- Does the patient need information in other formats? Some people find it hard to understand spoken information and may prefer either written information or the use of pictures.

- Would a referral to speech and language therapy be helpful? They are often trained in using Talking Mats, which is a tool to help people with verbal communication difficulties to communicate effectively.

- Is this the right time of day for asking the patient questions? If you know that your patient is much more drowsy in the morning than the afternoon, then ask the questions in the afternoon!

- One person should be asking the questions. If too many people become involved, the person could feel overwhelmed and more confused with all of the information.

- Distractions in the ward should be minimised.

Using the two-stage test, we can determine whether Sarah has capacity to make this decision (see Table 4.1).

Table 4.1: The Mental Capacity Act two-stage test

Two-stage test	Sarah
1) Is there an impairment of or disturbance in the functioning of the person's mind or brain (such as dementia, learning disabilities, schizophrenia)?	Sarah has dementia and she is currently described as confused.
2) Is the impairment or disturbance sufficient that the person lacks the capacity to make that particular decision? For stage 2, the person is unable to make a decision if they are unable to do one or more of the following things: • Understand the information relevant to the decision. • Retain the information for long enough to be able to make a decision. • Use or weigh up the information as part of the process of making the decision. • Communicate the decision by any possible method (talking, sign language, squeezing someone's hand).	Understanding: Does Sarah understand the information being discussed? Does she understand the need to stay in hospital and receive treatment and care? Does she understand the risks of going home without treatment? Retain: Can Sarah hold on to the information discussed long enough to make an informed decision? Use or weigh up: Is Sarah able to use the information discussed to make an informed decision? Can she weigh up the pros and cons of leaving hospital and refusing treatment? Communicate: Can Sarah make her feelings and wishes known about whether or not she wants to stay in hospital and receive care and treatment?

BEST INTERESTS

All decisions made for a person need to be in their best interests. Acting or making a decision in the best interests of a person who lacks capacity to make a decision is a well-established principle in common law, which is now set out in the Mental Capacity Act.

The only exceptions to this are around those who lack capacity participating in research and advance decisions to refuse treatment where other safeguards apply. It is impossible to give a single description of what best interests are since they depend almost entirely on individual circumstances. Normally, a person would use their own ideas of what is morally and ethically acceptable to make decisions but these ideas may not be shared with the other individuals involved in the decision-making process.

As professionals making the decisions for the person, we have no way of knowing exactly what the patient would have wanted in the circumstance unless a decision had been made before the loss of capacity. The professional has to find a way of acting with maximum consideration for the patient's needs and views, and this can sometimes be difficult.

For Sarah, we know that she has her partner and friends. These are the people who know her best. It was not possible to talk to her partner, but her friends gave staff a sense of what her previous views and wishes may have been.

If Sarah had no friends or family, it might have been necessary to instruct an independent mental capacity advocate (IMCA) to support her. The advocate's role is to represent a person in the decision-making process and ensure that the Mental Capacity Act is followed. Each hospital will have a list of local IMCAs.

RESTRAINT

At the start of the chapter, we looked at the paternalistic view that Sarah needs treatment and therefore we should ensure that she receives it, by whatever means possible. There are occasions when patients like Sarah will require a degree of restraint to facilitate treatment. When asked if they 'restrain' patients, most general hospital staff will fervently deny it. This shows a degree of ignorance about restraint, which is necessary and right as often as it is disproportionate and wrong. The most important thing about restraint is to understand it, use it correctly and ensure that everyone is supported fully during the process.

WHAT IS RESTRAINT?

Restraint happens when a person 'restricts a person's freedom of movement, whether they are resisting or not' (Mental Capacity Act 2005). It is important to remember that whether a person is being restrained or not does not depend on whether the person is consenting or not.

THE REGULATION OF RESTRAINT

A patient who is deemed to have mental capacity cannot be legally restrained against their will unless that person is being treated under the Mental Health Act or in dire emergencies under common law. Therefore, before restraint is considered, staff must be aware of whether the patient has capacity or not to make the decision required. If the person lacks capacity, the Mental Capacity Act is clear about how restraint should be used. These conditions must be satisfied in order to justify the use of restraint.

- The person using it believes it is necessary to *prevent harm* to Sarah.

- The degree of the restraint is *proportionate* to the degree of harm.

> If Sarah has capacity, she is allowed to make an unwise decision – you cannot restrain her because you do not agree with it.

- The *least restrictive option* must always be used.

- If restraint is necessary to prevent harm to the person who lacks capacity, it must be the minimum amount of force for the shortest time possible (Department of Constitutional Affairs 2007).

- The reason for the restraint and the evidence of regular review must be clearly documented.

Restraint is an area that is, by necessity, highly regulated. The clinician must understand the main principles of regulation and ensure that they are being adhered to. It is important to note also that the person who is actually restraining the patient is the person responsible and they must understand the consequences of their actions. Knowledge of these key areas will support the clinician to act legally.

RESTRAINT AND PEOPLE LIVING WITH DEMENTIA

In Sarah's case, the use of restraint is further complicated by the presence of her dementia and her previous lifestyle choices. Research has shown that the use of restraint in people with dementia is associated with negative physical outcomes (Evans, Wood and Lambert 2003) and that its use is often accompanied by feelings of shame, loss of dignity, self-respect, loss of identity, anxiety, aggression, isolation and disillusionment (Gallinagh et al. 2001).

Further considerations are identified in the box.

Issues with restraint in people with dementia

- Increased confusion in a delirium-prone group.

- A significant amount of challenging behaviour is purposeful – restraint of a patient might take away the ability of the patient to express an unmet need.

- If something is taken away from a person with dementia (such as removing a walking stick or use of hands with mittens), the person might forget how to use it afterwards.

Therefore, restraint for patients with dementia should only be used 'as a measure of last resort once all other approaches to manage a situation have been tried and found to have failed' (Hughes 2010).

WHAT ARE THE DIFFERENT TYPES OF RESTRAINT?

Any intentional restriction of a person's freedom of movement constitutes restraint; however, types of restraint can be divided into four broad categories: physical, chemical, environmental and positional. Any restraint used must be an evidence-based intervention. Restraints commonly used for people with dementia are:

- *Chemical restraint* – used to reduce agitation. Staff must follow NICE guidance and ensure the doses are proportionate.

- *Bedrails* – often used to stop agitated patients getting out of bed. Bedrails are effective to stop a person rolling out of bed, but not to use as a restraint to stop a person who wants to get out of bed (National Patient Safety Agency 2005). If the person is trying to get out of bed, raised rails can cause greater injury.

DEPRIVATION OF LIBERTY SAFEGUARDS

The Mental Capacity Act Deprivation of Liberty (MCA DOL) safeguards were introduced in 2007 (Department of Health 2007). The safeguards apply to anyone:

- aged 18 and over

- who suffers from a mental disorder or disability of the mind – such as dementia or a profound learning disability

- who lacks the capacity to give informed consent to the arrangements made for their care

- for whom deprivation of liberty (within the meaning of Article 5 of the European Convention on Human Rights) is considered after an independent assessment to be necessary in their best interests to protect them from harm.

WHAT IS DEPRIVATION OF LIBERTY?

A recent court decision has provided a definition of what is meant by the term 'deprivation of liberty'. A deprivation of liberty occurs when 'the person is under continuous supervision and control and is not free to leave, and the person lacks capacity to consent to these arrangements' (United Kingdom Supreme Court 2014).

It can be helpful to think of restrictions of a person's activity as being on a scale, from minimum restrictions at one end to the more extreme restrictions – deprivations of liberty – at the other end. One large restriction could in itself be a deprivation of liberty (such as sedating a person for non-medical reasons) or many small restrictions could combine to create a deprivation of liberty. There have been several test cases in the European Court of Human Rights and in the UK that have clarified which situations may constitute a deprivation of liberty:

- A patient being restrained in order to admit them to hospital.

- Medication being given against a person's will.

- Staff having complete control over a patient's care or movements for a long period.

- Staff making all decisions about a patient, including choices about assessments, treatment and visitors.

- Staff deciding whether a patient can be released into the care of others or to live elsewhere.

- Staff refusing to discharge a person into the care of others.

- Staff restricting a person's access to their friends or family.

(Alzheimer's Society 2012)

If Sarah is found to lack capacity, a decision will be made in her best interests to keep her in hospital and to treat her. Sarah wants to go home to her partner, but that is currently unsafe and therefore she will be restrained if she tries to leave. If this restraint continues for several days, then it is necessary to apply for a Deprivation of Liberties Safeguards Assessment. Where the care/treatment plan for an individual lacking capacity will unavoidably result in a deprivation of liberty judged to be in that person's best interests, this *must* be authorised (United Kingdom Supreme Court 2014).

LASTING POWER OF ATTORNEY

It is recognised that there are times in a person's life when they might not be able to make a decision. This might be because the person has advanced dementia or because a person has become unable to express their own wishes. If the person has made provision in advance, the responsibility for making decisions can be passed on to a nominated individual. This is called giving someone Lasting Power of Attorney (LPA).

In the England and Wales, there are two kinds of LPA:

- *Personal welfare*, which is about making decisions around health and medical care. It might also include decisions about going into a care home.

- *Property and affairs*, which allows the nominated person to make financial decisions.

The nominated individual can only make decisions pertaining to the type of LPA that they hold. The LPA must be arranged and ratified when the person still has the mental capacity to agree to the decision and it can only be activated when the person is deemed to lack capacity for a decision.

For an LPA to be legal, it must be registered with the Office of the Public Guardian. The person holding the LPA must be able to show documentary evidence of this before a clinician accepts that there is an LPA in place.

There are limitations in the scope of decisions that a nominated person can make even with an LPA. For health and welfare, decisions can be made on:

- daily routines such as washing, dressing and eating

- medical care

- living arrangements.

However, the nominated person is not permitted to make a decision about keeping the person alive unless it is specifically stated in the Lasting Power of Attorney document. This will continue to be the decision of the senior clinician unless the person has an Advanced Directive, Living Will or Priorities of Care in place (see Chapter 14).

In Scotland

A similar system is operated. There are three types of Power of Attorney (POA):

- *Continuing* for financial and property affairs
- *Welfare* for health and care decisions
- *Combined* for both.

How to make best practice happen

Have I asked why Sarah is reacting this way?	Sarah is upset about what has happened and misses her partner; she does not understand why she is being kept separate from him as she has chosen to stay in the past after fights – Sarah's anger with her situation is a normal reaction.	
What are Sarah's strengths/ abilities?	Sarah is able to make many of her own decisions and voice her needs clearly. Sarah is independently mobile and can manage her personal hygiene.	
	Qualified staff	**Healthcare support worker**
Am I listening?	What does Sarah say when you try to deliver care or stop her from leaving?	Listen to Sarah; she is obviously angry because she's being kept from her loved one. Imagine being kept from the person you love, even in such circumstances.
Do I know enough about Sarah?	Sarah's friends can help to explain her home situation and a little about what Sarah likes.	What can you find out about Sarah from her and her friends? Don't judge the situation on your own beliefs and feelings.
What can I do to enable Sarah?	Give Sarah time to explain herself; do not dismiss what she is saying. Even though Sarah is being treated in her best interests, it is important to remember that she can make her own decisions about other things and to encourage her to do this as much as possible.	If Sarah becomes angry and agitated, listen to her thoughts and feelings, empathising with why she feels that way. Discuss her life with her partner, focusing on happier times. Let Sarah keep control of as much as possible and give her choice wherever you can.

Chapter 5

Patrick – Communication

Patrick is 77 years old and was diagnosed with Alzheimer's disease three years ago. He is known to his friends as Paddy and is a widower, having lost his wife 20 years ago. Paddy is fully independent and attends his local memory cafe once a week. Dementia has never really interfered with his daily life and he uses strategies like his iPhone to support his memory. He jokes, 'I carry my memory in my pocket.' He is proud that he is managing so well.

Paddy fell over and broke his glasses while walking to a taxi this evening. He felt unwell earlier today and consumed a few glasses of wine with his meal. Paramedics took him to the emergency department and on arrival Paddy is unable to answer any questions on his medical or life history.

HOW DEMENTIA AFFECTS COMMUNICATION

Communication is particularly important in hospital where patients can feel vulnerable, alone and frightened. We need to consider how we communicate with our patients, and we also need to have skills in recognising what is being communicated to us to ensure that we provide the highest-quality care.

As we age, we will experience changes to our senses, including hearing and vision. These will impact on our ability to communicate, particularly in the case of Paddy as his glasses were broken in the fall. He came into hospital unable to read and was having difficulty seeing his immediate environment, making his world very confusing.

A person with dementia's ability to communicate is based on the progression of the disease but also the individual's personal resources. Paddy had been functioning at a very high level in the community despite being diagnosed with dementia three years ago, but when he was admitted to hospital he seemed to deteriorate very quickly from his baseline. The impact of his illness and the admission had a significant and detrimental effect on his level of functioning and this is a common experience for many people with dementia.

Communication can be hampered by barriers that lead to misunderstandings, resentments, frustrations and demoralisation not only for patients, but also for staff. It is important to be aware of what those barriers are and to work with the person and their family to overcome them.

BARRIERS TO COMMUNICATION EXPERIENCED BY PEOPLE WITH DEMENTIA: APHASIA

This can affect a person's ability to communicate. The person can hear what is being said, but damage to the brain causes it to be misinterpreted and as a consequence they may:

- not understand what other people say and they may feel as though others are talking in an unknown foreign language

- not understand when people speak in long, complex sentences and may forget the start of the sentence

- not understand others if there is background noise or if different people are talking in a group.

Other problems include:

- Word-finding difficulties and using 'empty phrases' such as 'that thing' or 'you know'.

- Reduced understanding.

- Changes to semantic memory. Semantic memory is a recollection of facts gathered when we are young – it is essentially common knowledge, such as knowing that grass is green.

- Repeating words and thoughts over and over.

- Using generalised descriptions of an object whose name they can't remember or using a substitute word or even a new word.

- Easily losing train of thought.

- Difficulty organising words logically.

- Writing and reading skills may also deteriorate.

- Reverting to first language.

- Saying very little and finding it particularly hard to initiate a conversation.

- Relying on gestures more than speaking.

- Perceptual difficulties.

- Changes to emotional state.

- Lower threshold for sensory overload.

STRESS RESPONSE TO A HOSPITAL ADMISSION

When Paddy was admitted, he was unable to give much information to the staff, who had locked his phone away as they did not want to lose it. Paddy was told this, but could not retain the information, so he spent the majority of his time getting out of bed to search for it and trying to leave. Paddy explained that he wanted to go home and became increasingly upset when he was stopped from going. This escalated to a point where the staff decided to sedate him. After this, he slept all day, missed his meals and was incontinent. His medical notes stated that he had 'advanced dementia' as a result of his deteriorated level of function and his behaviour. Paddy was also diagnosed as having a hyperactive delirium.

John, Paddy's son, had been away and contacted the ward on day five; he was shocked by the change in his father since the week before when they had spoken via Skype.

When people like Paddy are acutely unwell, it can be a real challenge for them to communicate their needs to staff. The combination of deteriorated cognition, low mood, a change in environment, pain and anxiety about bothering staff can all create blocks to communication.

WAYS TO SUPPORT GOOD COMMUNICATION

Some of us are naturally adept at communicating and others find it more challenging, but it is a skill that can be honed and developed over time. It is important to reflect back on interactions with others and consider what works well and what can be improved; keeping a reflective diary may be beneficial.

The key to good communication is the understanding that it is a two-way interaction and relies as much on hearing what is being conveyed as transmitting information effectively. Patients like Paddy need to be supported to maximise their communication skills.

There are five main ways that we communicate (see Figure 5.1).

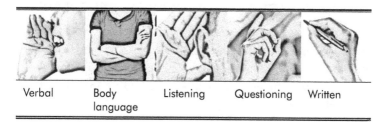

| Verbal | Body language | Listening | Questioning | Written |

Figure 5.1: Five ways that we communicate

We need to hear what our patients are saying and work out what it really means. The best way to do this is to remain quiet and encourage the patient to speak with gentle head nodding and, when appropriate, positive words and simple questions. Paddy responded well to having his hand held (see Chapter 15).

Try to identify the emotions behind the words; this can be particularly helpful if it is difficult to follow the content of a conversation. When the patient has finished speaking, reflect back to them about what you have understood. This shows that you are listening and being attentive, and the person has an opportunity to correct you.

It is also important to think about the questions that we ask. Cambridge University Hospitals NHS Foundation Trust's *Brief Encounters* (2014) explains that open questions encourage the person to respond freely with their thoughts and feelings, whereas closed questions classically produce one-word answers, such as 'yes' or 'no', which provide limited information.

Questions which start with 'what', 'where', 'which', 'who' and 'when', 'in what way' are open and will allow the person to respond in more detail. These will generate more interesting and thought-provoking answers. Table 5.1 shows the difference between an open and a closed question.

Table 5.1: Closed versus open question

Closed question	Open question
Are you hungry?	What are your favourite foods?

As well as listening and engaging in conversation you will also need to observe behaviour, as non-verbal communication will provide you with a considerable amount of information about a person's well-being. This will be touched on in many of the other chapters.

DIFFERENT REALITIES

It is not unusual for a person with dementia to believe something that is different from their current reality – for example, that they are younger or that dead relatives are still alive.

This often happens when a person is in hospital and can be seen as a stress response as well as a form of communication. By expressing a need to see a long-dead mother or father, for example, the person is expressing a need for safety and security.

For many years, this was treated like a delusion or hallucination whereby the clinician would correct the person and try to orientate them to reality. However, it was ineffective as it failed to address the need being communicated by the person.

VALIDATION

Validation therapy advocates that, rather than trying to bring the person with dementia back to our reality, it is more positive to enter their reality. In this way empathy is developed with the person, building trust and a sense of security. This in turn reduces anxiety.

Some carers express concern that validation involves lying to the person with dementia about reality. However, a more accurate description is that it avoids challenging their reality. For instance, if a person with dementia believes that she is waiting for her children (who are all now middle-aged) to return from school, carers who use a validation approach would not argue the point or expect their relative to have insight into their behaviour. They would not correct their beliefs. Rather, the validating approach proposes acknowledging and empathising with the feelings behind the behaviour being expressed. In this way the person's dignity and self-esteem are maintained.

A helpful approach and an aid to memory when working with patients diagnosed with dementia is VERA (Validate, Emotion, Reassure, Activity) (Blackhall *et al.* 2011). When

Paddy was trying to leave the ward, he told staff he wanted to go to his wife who had died many years ago. Table 5.2 illustrates how effective the VERA approach can be.

Table 5.2: Using VERA to support Paddy

Validate	Accepting that the behaviour exhibited has a value to the person and is not just a symptom of dementia.
	'You sound really worried, Paddy; tell me about your wife and children.'
	Here you accept Paddy's perception of the problem, you don't question, and you encourage him to say more.
Emotion	Paying attention to the emotional content of what the person is saying.
	'Your wife and children clearly mean the world to you, Paddy.'
	This shows that you understand the love he has for his wife and children.
Reassure	Can be as simple as saying 'It'll be okay' and smiling or holding their hand.
	'Paddy, your son, John, called earlier and he said that he will be coming to see you on Saturday, when he flies in from Australia.'
	This will reassure Paddy, and help him to re-orientate to the present.
Activity	People with dementia need to feel occupied and active, so see if you can engage them in some related activity.
	'Let's have a look at the photo album your friend brought in yesterday, I remember you saying that there are some lovely pictures of your son and daughter-in-law and grandchildren.'
	This activity fits in with Paddy's preoccupation with his family, and incorporates his behaviour rather than invalidating it.

Communication as a theme resonates throughout this book. Good communication is essential for any clinician caring for people with dementia.

TOP COMMUNICATION TIPS FOR CLINICIANS

These top tips provide an excellent framework to support good communication:

- *Gain attention.* Gain the listener's attention before you begin talking. Approach the person from the front, identify yourself and call him or her by their preferred name. Make eye contact, try and be at their eye level with them, use gentle touch (if appropriate) and smile.

- *Consider the message.* What do you want to say and how you will say it? Always approach your patients in a calm manner, even if you have a million and one things to do. Our patients will pick up on our stress, and they may choose not to engage with you as they could think you are too busy.

- *Minimise distractions.* Ensure that the person can see and hear you and try to reduce background noise. It may be helpful to pull the curtains around the bed so that you can have the patient's full attention.

- *Make the most of relatives.* Ask for advice from family/main carers about the best way to communicate with the patient.

- *Be attentive.* Show that you are listening and search for meaning. Repeat what you think the patient means and seek confirmation.

- *Speak naturally.* Speak at a normal rate – not too fast or too slow. Use pauses to give the person time to process what you're saying. Use short, simple and familiar phrases (such as 'spend a penny').

- *Be concise.* Give one-step directions and ask only one question at a time. Identify people and things by name, avoiding pronouns, and offer simple choices.

- *Be specific.* Use accessible, unambiguous language.

- *Be positive.* Instead of saying, 'Don't do that,' say, 'Let's try this.'

- *Repeat and/or rephrase as necessary.* If the patient has difficulty understanding what you're saying, find a different way of saying it.

- *Be patient.* Encourage the person to continue to express their thoughts, even if they are having difficulty. Ensure that the patient has enough time and does not feel rushed, and that your non-verbal communication (for example, facial expression and posture) is friendly and patient. Be careful not to interrupt and avoid criticising, correcting and arguing.

- *Use non-verbal communication.* Use this as much as possible, including gestures, visual prompts and cues. Observe all non-verbal communication and check its message (for example, a person may not understand, but nods to be polite) and encourage the patient to use non-verbal communication, including visual prompts, demonstrations and body language.

- *Use communications aids.* Consider the use of further communication aids, such as talking mats. Ensure that the patient has their hearing aid, that it is switched on and the battery is working. Writing messages down for patients on small whiteboards or paper can be helpful. If the patient is non-English speaking, you can learn and use some words and phrases that are meaningful and relevant to them or ask the family or friends to write down statements that can be read out to the patient.

(Adapted from *Advice for Nurses and Other Healthcare Professionals*, Alzheimer's Society 2014)

How to make best practice happen

Have I asked why Paddy is reacting this way?	Paddy's mobile phone was extremely important to him as a means of communication with his friends and family, and he also relied on it as his 'memory'.
	Paddy does not understand where his phone has gone and is looking for it.
	The loss of his phone has unsettled him.
What are Paddy's strengths/ abilities?	Paddy is able to use technology to support his day-to-day life. Enabling him to continue using this while he is in hospital will help to retain his skills. Paddy is close to his son and lives independently.

	Qualified staff	**Healthcare support worker**
Am I listening?	Paddy is telling you that he is unhappy and unsettled through his behaviour. Think about how he communicates at home – are you giving him the means to do this in hospital (phone/ glasses)?	What is Paddy telling you with his behaviour? Have you made it possible for him to communicate to you?
Do I know enough about Paddy?	Paddy relies heavily on his mobile phone. Ask the son to complete a 'This is Me' document (it can be emailed). What can the son tell you about Paddy's interests?	Paddy relies on his phone to support him living independently. Appreciate this and ensure that Paddy has his phone. Familiarise yourself with the 'This is Me' document; engage with Paddy about his life, discussing experiences, family and past hobbies.

	Qualified staff	**Healthcare support worker**
What can I do to enable Paddy?	Ask the family to complete a 'This is Me' document, to help staff get to know Paddy and what is important to him. Take time to be with Paddy and try to understand what he is trying to communicate. Give Paddy his phone back and ask a friend to bring his tablet in.	Ensure that Paddy has access to his phone and tablet at all times, making sure that he can charge them close to his bed. Discuss with Paddy how he has become so competent using technology. Engage with Paddy about things that are important to him.

Chapter 6

John – Physical Health Needs

John has been admitted to hospital after a fall at home. He has a background of osteoporosis, dementia, diabetes and recurrent falls. He lives alone in a house and until recently has been fully independent in all his activities of daily living. John has been admitted to hospital on three occasions in the past eight weeks. Two admissions were after he became hypoglycaemic and one was from a fall. Paramedics have documented that John's flat was very unkempt, there was no food in the fridge and there were piles of unused medication lying around the house. When the doctor asked John what medication he usually takes, John was unable to tell the doctor. It is evident that John is struggling to cope at home.

John is an avid reader and has told staff that he loves reading so much he even 'reads the back of cereal boxes'.

FRAILTY

An increasing number of people with dementia live with frailty. Frailty is a syndrome which is more common in older people, affecting 25–50 per cent of those over the age of 80 years (British Geriatrics Society 2014). The British Geriatrics Society describes frailty as 'a distinctive health state related to the ageing process in which multiple body systems gradually lose their in-built reserves'. There are different models to describe frailty, which fall into two broad categories (see Table 6.1).

Table 6.1: The different models of frailty

Phenotype	Deficit model
Describes characteristics such as weight loss, reduced muscle strength, reduced gait, speed, exhaustion or low energy. Three or more of these together would indicate frailty.	Looks at an accumulation of deficits such as loss of hearing, low mood, tremor or diseases such as dementia. These contribute to a matrix of frailty.

Because of their lack of reserves, people with frailty are more likely to have serious outcomes from a relatively minor event, such as an infection or a fall. People with frailty are also at very high risk of developing delirium when they are in hospital.

It is important to identify a patient who is frail or at risk of frailty to ensure that care is tailored towards preventing deterioration and modifying any risk factors if they are present. John's increasing frailty led to multiple admissions and this would escalate until his frailty needs were addressed.

FALLS

People with dementia suffer more falls, more fractures and higher post-fracture mortality than those without dementia, yet they are under-assessed for risk factors for falls and are less likely to receive treatment for osteoporosis (Menzies *et al.* 2010). In Chapter 2, we spoke about the importance of gathering relevant information in order to understand the individual; this includes information on how the patient is normally able to walk or get from their bed to the toilet or their armchair. Staff must consider fear of falling as well as being mindful of what the patient can achieve or believes that they can achieve.

Assistive technology such as bed sensors, low-rise beds and falls alarms can support the prevention of falls in the busy ward environment.

Strategies to increase the safety of those at risk of falling:

- Ensure that the individual wears non-slip socks.

- Ensure that the individual's mobility aid is near their hand.

- Demonstrate the use of the call bell and reinforce its use as often as necessary.

- Provide regular prompts to the individual on the location of the toilet.

- Remove all clutter and tripping hazards.

- Orientate the patient to the environment in detail appropriate to their sensory/cognitive faculties.

- Educate the patient on any strategies introduced to prevent falls.

- Ensure that the patient has their appropriate sensory aids (glasses, hearing aids).

CONTINENCE

On admission, John's clothes were dirty and smelled of urine. He had been trying to get to the toilet when he fell and had been incontinent of urine. This led to an assumption that he was incontinent and a pad was put on him, leading to further episodes of incontinence while on the ward.

Incontinence is not an inevitable consequence of dementia; however, dementia can cause people to experience episodes of incontinence for various reasons. During early and mild stages of dementia, many problems leading to incontinence are manageable (Waite *et al.* 2009). Prior to coming into hospital, John was not incontinent; however, we can see how various factors contributed to this, including:

- unfamiliar environment

- increased confusion

- reduced mobility

- visual and auditory impairments.

If a patient experiences incontinence at some point in their stay, it is important not to assume they are incontinent while at home. It is good practice to support patients by implementing management strategies that reduce the risk of incontinence. Strategies can include:

- Avoid caffeinated drinks as they can act as bladder stimulants.

- Regularly orientate the patient to the toilet and bathrooms.

- Ensure that patients are provided with adequate assistance to get to the toilet in time.

- Ensure that there is adequate signage for the bathroom, using both words and pictures.

- Provide bedpans or commodes at the bedside for patients who are less mobile but continent.

- Understand that patients may not be expressing a need for the toilet and so remind and prompt them regularly (two to three hourly).

- Remember that patients may express their need for the toilet in other less obvious ways, such as wandering or trying to climb out of bed, so try to pick up on what these are for each patient.

- Consider using familiar phrases such as 'spend a penny' when encouraging patients to use the toilet.

- Provide assistance if patients have difficulty completing the sequence of actions required to go to the toilet, such as removing clothes or recognising the toilet.

Incontinence aids should only be used with patients who are known to be incontinent before admission. The use of incontinence aids with patients who are normally continent can lead to permanent loss of continence. For many people with dementia, the loss of continence can be the final straw which precipitates admission into a care setting. Hospital staff must prioritise continence, as getting it wrong for a person like John can have a dramatic and negative impact for the rest of his life.

VISION AND DEMENTIA

People with dementia may experience changes in their sight that cause them to misinterpret the world around them. They can have healthy eyes but visual difficulties caused by changes in the brain. A healthy brain interprets what the eyes see, and to do this it also uses the other senses, thoughts, feelings and memories. When a person becomes aware of what they have seen, it is then perceived and interpreted. It is quite a complex process which can be affected by damage to the brain. In people with dementia, this often leads to visuoperceptual changes.

These can also occur as part of the normal ageing process, but there are specific dementias that can directly impact on vision such as Lewy Body, Posterior Cortical Atrophy, Alzheimer's disease and vascular dementia.

Visuoperceptual changes are under-diagnosed in people with dementia because the signs can be difficult to separate from other symptoms. One condition may mask or be mistaken for the effects of the other and lead to inaction. Common difficulties include:

- reading
- recognising people
- coping with changes in light – from bright to low lights or vice versa
- finding things
- avoiding obstacles
- recognising food and drink.

Unusual behaviour may be a reaction to sight loss or an attempt to maximise useful vision. In an unfamiliar environment a person with visuoperceptual difficulties might:

- become withdrawn or uncommunicative
- be clumsy or falling
- report visual hallucinations
- hold items up close
- be more confused and disorientated
- be startled by noises or people approaching.

John should have his regular glasses with him, and they should be clean and functional. If they have been lost, the ward should have a small supply of inexpensive glasses to lend patients. It is also important to ensure that there is good lighting when John is trying to do anything and that he is cared for in a clutter-free environment to help him navigate more easily.

If the patient is experiencing problems with sight, then they should be seen by an optician, who will be able to provide eye tests with some reasonable adjustments. It may be possible to refer them to specialist services while they are an in-patient. Many opticians also offer home services and some have additional dementia training to support patients like John who might find it difficult to go out to an optician.

HEARING AND DEMENTIA

It is estimated that nine million people in the UK are deaf or hard of hearing, and this number is rising as people live longer. There is a significant increase in the proportion of deaf people from around the age of 50, and by 70 over 71 per cent of the population is deaf or has significant hearing loss, so it is likely that the majority of older patients will have some hearing impairment. When caring for John, we need to remember this and not assume that his unresponsiveness relates to his dementia.

Staff can check with John or his family to determine the best way to communicate and ensure that any hearing aids are in use and functioning.

Communication with a person who is deaf can be maximised if the clinician approaches the patient in the right way. Helpful ways of doing this include:

- Choose a quiet place or minimise background noise.

- Get the patient's attention before you start speaking.

- Make sure they can see your face clearly; do not cover your mouth.

- Get yourself at eye level with them.

- Do not shout or raise your voice; this will distort your speech, making it difficult to understand.

- Say clearly what the conversation is about.

- Keep the message simple.

- Speak a little more slowly than usual.

- Do not over-exaggerate your words as you speak.

- If the patient is having difficulty understanding, try another word to express your meaning.

- Use gestures to back up what you mean.

- Try writing things down.

Deaf people rely on visual cues, so ensure that the patient has clean and appropriate prescription glasses, if appropriate.

ORAL HEALTH

John's mouth was dirty and he had oral thrush which impacted on his ability to eat and drink, increasing his frailty. John's problems with oral hygiene might have been because of his frailty, such as struggling to stand at a sink and clean his teeth, or he might have been forgetting to clean his teeth because of his cognitive impairment. The impact of good oral health has been outlined in a recent report by the British Dental Association (2013):

- *Quality of life:* to allow people to continue to talk comfortably and confidently, enjoy eating, maintain confidence in their appearance and be pain-free.

- *Medical reasons:* to manage the side-effects of medications taken for dementia and its symptoms, maintain adequate nutrition and minimise sources of micro-organisms that may later involve other parts of the body such as aspiration into the lungs (aspiration pneumonia is a common cause of death in patients with Alzheimer's disease).

- *Dental reasons:* to prevent the development of dental problems, complications and emergencies or the need for general anaesthesia and to minimise the risk of unnecessary tooth extractions.

- *Behavioural problems:* behavioural problems that are caused by dental pain can be minimised with good oral health. Such problems include a disinterest in or avoidance of food, pulling at the mouth or face, chewing of the lip or tongue, excessive grinding.

PROBLEMS WITH MAINTAINING ORAL HEALTH

Research has shown that people with dementia are more likely to have poor oral hygiene, tooth decay, poor gingival health and more non-functional teeth. People with dentures who have dementia are less likely to take them out at night and less likely to remember to clean them (BDA 2013). Key interventions for John would be:

- Check his mouth, to ensure that there are no mouth ulcers or rotten teeth that might be causing pain.

- Ensure that his dentures are kept with him and kept clean.

- Help John to clean his remaining teeth twice daily.

- Encourage John to drink some water after eating sugary foods.

DIABETES AND DEMENTIA

People with type 2 diabetes are at higher risk of developing dementia than those without diabetes. As diabetic care is focused around self-management, there can be challenges for a person with cognitive impairment when it comes to managing the condition. John was forgetting to self-administer drugs and then taking more than one dose at a time because of his memory impairment which caused his diabetes to become uncontrolled. Below are some of the recommended approaches for supporting a person with dementia who has diabetes:

- Support self-care (or care given by their partner) as long as possible (for example, testing blood, glucose, injecting insulin). Review self-care ability regularly.

- Ask the GP to simplify medication regimes and tablet load, preferably once daily. Ask the pharmacist about tools to support self-medication such as blister packs and timed 'dosset' boxes.

- Be vigilant about behaviour change as the symptoms of diabetes or the complications of diabetes may be ignored and assumed to be personality traits. Loud aggression may be a symptom of low blood glucose, for example.

- Meals should be provided in a calm and distraction-free environment.

- Encourage a nourishing diet that provides sufficient calories to maintain ideal weight and fits the person's usual meal pattern.

How to make best practice happen

Have I asked why John is reacting this way?	John is frail and has become unable to cope at home independently.	
What are John's strengths/ abilities?	John is used to being independent and doing things for himself John likes to read and reads well.	
	Qualified staff	**Healthcare support worker**
Am I listening?	What things are important to John to keep doing? There might be some areas that he does not mind receiving help for but others where he is keen to be independent.	Listen to physiotherapy and occupational therapy assessments to find out what John is capable of doing himself. Ask John what he wants to do.
Do I know enough about John?	Talk to John about how he lived before he was older and what he reads. Try to tailor his care and discharge plan to his interests and needs. Encourage him or his family to fill in a 'This is Me' document and make sure staff are familiar with it.	Use John's love of books to start a conversation, read his 'This is Me' document with him and talk about the content while helping him.

What can I do to enable John?	Use the many things that John can do to support the areas where he is a little weaker.	Do not do things for John if he can do them himself – even if it takes longer to complete a task.
	Ensure that John's routine on the ward is as close as possible to his home routine.	You might want to consider writing down instructions for tasks for him.
	Make sure the ward staff are aware that they need to encourage him to be as independent as possible.	Remember that John is continent – assist him to safely use the ward toilets, commode or urine bottles as instructed.
	Use John's ability to read to support his independence. For example, can his medication instructions be written down in a way that would enable him to take them at the right times?	Remind John to use his glasses, hearing aid and dentures and help to keep them clean.
		If John is able to test his own blood glucose, try to get someone to bring in his own testing kit so he can continue to do it himself. If you are assisting him with testing, involve him in the action and engage with him about what you are doing and why.

Chapter 7

Jaheem – Delirium

> Jaheem is 72 years old and was diagnosed with Alzheimer's disease eight months ago. He lives with his wife and adult son, and manages without any support. He works twice a week in the office of the family construction firm. He has been admitted as an elective patient for a trans urethral resection of the prostate (TURP). The surgery went well; however, yesterday it was noted that he was in a bad mood and he refused therapy input, stating he 'wants to sleep instead'. He has accused a member of staff of stealing something from him and he pulled out his urinary catheter which had to be replaced in a painful procedure. Last night he became aggressive with staff and kept trying to leave. This morning he is calm again but expressing paranoid ideas and asking to go home.

WHAT IS DELIRIUM?

Delirium is described by the National Institute for Health and Care Excellence (NICE) to be an 'acute confusional state' and is a clinical syndrome characterised by disturbed consciousness, cognitive function or perception which has an acute onset and fluctuating course (NICE 2010). It can occur in any setting, but is a common consequence of hospital admission in older patients. Up to 30 per cent of patients in medical wards and as many as 50 per cent of people post-surgery will develop delirium (Healthcare Improvement Scotland 2014). If a person has a pre-existing dementia, they are five times more likely to get delirium.

Patients who get delirium have higher morbidity and mortality rates, longer hospital stays and are more likely to have a functional decline afterwards. The underlying cause of the delirium might also be a physiological event such as a pulmonary embolism or a cardiac event. It is therefore important to recognise it, identify the cause and treat it as a medical emergency.

Delirium is usually a short-term state, which resolves when the cause has been treated. The average duration can be hours to weeks. It has been suggested that in some patients, it can persist for months but that is unusual. It can present in different ways:

Hyperactive – increased motor activity, agitation, hallucinations and inappropriate behaviour.

Hypoactive – reduced motor activity and lethargy. This is more common in older people, has a poorer prognosis and is frequently missed.

Mixed – a combination of both types.

The fluctuations in Jaheem's alertness and activity suggested that he had a mixed delirium.

WHAT ARE THE RISK FACTORS?

Patients like Jaheem are at higher risk of developing delirium, because of specific risk factors (see Figure 7.1).

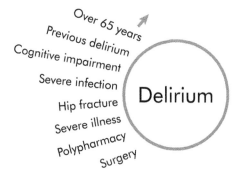

Figure 7.1: Risk factors for delirium

TRIGGERS

An episode of delirium can be triggered by a particular event or stressor. Jaheem had several risk factors (cognitive impairment, age and recent surgery) and triggers (immobility, bladder catheter). However, any small event might have triggered an episode of delirium. The main triggers are identified below:

- immobility
- critical illness
- use of physical restraint
- bladder catheters
- iatrogenic events (such as a pulmonary embolism or a hospital acquired infection)
- malnutrition
- psychoactive medication
- dehydration
- intercurrent illness.

INTERVENTIONS TO PREVENT DELIRIUM

Evidence has shown that if patients who are at high risk of developing delirium are managed appropriately, the risk of developing it can be significantly reduced (see Table 7.1).

Table 7.1: Prevention of delirium in high-risk patients (NICE 2010)

Avoid	Try
Cognitive impairment or disorientation	Active orientation, visible clocks and signage, stimulating activities, regular visits from family and friends.
Dehydration or constipation	Encourage person to drink. Actively manage risk of constipation and/or treat existing constipation.
Hypoxia	Assess for hypoxia and optimise oxygen saturation.
Immobility or limited mobility	Encourage early mobilisation after surgery and mobilisation in all groups.
Infection	Look for and treat infection. Avoid urinary catheters.
Multiple medications	Carry out a medication review, rationalising medications where clinically appropriate.
Pain	Assess for pain using an appropriate tool (see Chapter 8).
Poor nutrition	Ensure that dentures are fitting well. Monitor dietary intake.
Sensory impairment	Ensure that reversible causes of impairment (such as earwax) are corrected. Ensure that the person has all sensory aids available and in use.
Sleep disturbance	Avoid interventions at night where possible, encourage good sleep hygiene and reduce daytime sleeping.

RECOGNITION OF DELIRIUM

Delirium is unrecognised by nurses and doctors in over 66 per cent of cases (NICE 2010). It is often mistaken for dementia and depression or not noticed at all if it is the hypoactive type. The NICE Delirium Pathway identified four indicators which suggest a person might have delirium (see Table 7.2). The key to these is to look for a *recent change*.

Table 7.2: Early signs of delirium

Change in cognitive function	Worsened concentration
	Slow responses
	Confusion
Perception changes	Visual hallucinations
	Auditory hallucinations
	Paranoia
Physical function changes	Reduced mobility and movement
	Restlessness/agitation
	Changes in appetite
	Sleep disturbance
Social behaviour changes	Lack of cooperation with reasonable requests
	Withdrawal
	Alterations in communication or attitude

If delirium is suspected, the patient will require a full assessment including investigations into the cause of the delirium. The Confusion Assessment Method is a validated tool that is routinely used and has a sensitivity of 94 per cent (Young and Inouye 2007).

The Confusion Assessment Method (CAM) Diagnostic Algorithm looks at four features:

- Feature 1: acute onset and fluctuating course

- Feature 2: inattention

- Feature 3: disorganised thinking

- Feature 4: altered level of consciousness.

The diagnosis of delirium by CAM requires the presence of features 1 and 2 and either 3 or 4. More recently, other tools have been developed which use the same principles, and the most commonly used of these is the 4AT (Healthcare Improvement Scotland 2014).

MANAGING DELIRIUM

Managing the needs of a person with delirium requires similar interventions to those that are used to prevent it.

Explain what is happening to Jaheem and his family

Experiencing delirium, either as a patient or a family member, can be very frightening; when that person already has dementia, there is often an assumption that the behaviour is because of the dementia and that the person will stay like that forever. It is important to help Jaheem and his family understand that this is an acute problem and that it is likely to resolve. The hospital should have leaflets about delirium, which can be given to Jaheem's family to help them understand it.

Identify and treat the cause

Delirium in hospital is often caused by a physical event, such as the development of sepsis, a myocardial infarction or a pulmonary embolism. These physical factors need to be tested for and ruled out to ensure that Jaheem is not being affected by a life-threatening condition.

The other, non-threatening causes, such as constipation, dehydration and lack of stimulation, must also be ruled out.

Minimise moves (especially at night)

Jaheem is already disorientated and agitated and this is worse at night when there are fewer cues and aids available to him. If he is moved into another ward, this will increase his disorientation and his paranoia about the staff, whom he will not know.

Maximise orientation

If Jaheem is helped to orientate himself to time and place and to understand what has happened to him, he will be less anxious and more able to cope with the situation. His family can assist by providing him with familiar objects from home and things that interest him. The staff can help by ensuring that he has a visible clock nearby, and information saying where he is. A small whiteboard or even a sheet of paper can be used to provide orientation.

Monitor intake

Because Jaheem is delirious, it is likely that he will lose interest in eating and drinking. It is also possible that he will become paranoid about the content of food and drink being offered and refuse it. This is why the risk of people developing dehydration and malnutrition when they are delirious is high, and staff need to closely monitor Jaheem's intake, taking action if it falls below an acceptable level.

Proactive pain management

Staff need to ensure that Jaheem's pain is properly assessed and managed. Pain is both a trigger and cause of prolonged delirium and therefore needs to be managed according to the strategies outlined in Chapter 8.

Stimulation and activity in the day

It is important to keep Jaheem mentally active. He needs to use his brain and also be occupied to prevent boredom. Encourage his family to help with this. Evidence suggests that the presence of a person's family shortens the duration of the delirium.

Good sleep hygiene

It is difficult to sleep in an acute hospital and Jaheem has started sleeping in the day. It is important for staff to ensure that he gets to sleep at night and stays awake during the day. There is a risk that his sleep/wake cycle (circadian cycle) will reverse and that he will stop sleeping at night altogether. This can be disastrous for a person with dementia and can result in that person requiring care home admission, as families are often unable to cope when this happens.

The key elements of good sleep hygiene are identified by Barulich, Rizzardi and Sunden (2012):

- Reduce noise and interruptions at night – minimise unnecessary observations and use quieter equipment such as silent closing bins. Reduce nursing footfall past beds.

- Avoid giving the patient stimulants such as coffee, tea or caffeine drinks in the evening.

- Establish a regular sleep pattern (in other words, trying to sleep at the same time every night).

- Provide assistive devices to help the patient reposition themselves in bed (these can be bedrails if it is safe to use them).

- Restrict daytime sleeping.

- Try to encourage physical activity in the day if the patient is well enough.

- Review the patient's medication to ensure that drugs which affect sleep are avoided.

- Consider the use of massage as it has been found to be a significant method of sleep promotion.

USE OF SEDATION IN DELIRIOUS PATIENTS

If a patient is very distressed or is a risk to themselves or others, a short-term course of antipsychotics might be indicated. This is a last resort and should be discussed with the family where available. Drugs should be administered according to the NICE guidance on delirium (NICE 2010). This recommends that patients with delirium are always started on low-dose medication which can be titrated according to need.

Remember that once the patient has been sedated they have an increased risk of falls/injury and will therefore require closer supervision.

How to make best practice happen

Have I asked why Jaheem is reacting this way?	Jaheem is acting this way because he is delirious.	
	Staff need to identify and treat the cause of his delirium.	
	Jaheem needs close observations and medical support until the cause of his delirium is identified and treated.	
What are Jaheem's strengths/ abilities?	Jaheem was physically active before being ill and was very interested in construction.	
	Jaheem likes being active and is used to being the person in the family who makes decisions.	
	Jaheem has very strong bonds with his family.	
	Qualified staff	**Healthcare support worker**
Am I listening?	Jaheem is anxious and is expressing this through anger and requests to go home. Try to identify what is making him anxious at that moment.	Do not disregard what Jaheem is saying because he has delirium. Listen to what he is saying to you and think about the emotions behind his words.

Do I know enough about Jaheem?	Find out what interests Jaheem and how he normally sleeps. Family can be asked to bring in favourite things. Jaheem was proud of his strength and was very much the master in his family.	Appreciate that Jaheem has his own routine and way of doing things. He likes to be in control and has old-fashioned views about men and women.
What can I do to enable Jaheem?	Plan care based on his ability to walk and his strength. Use his interest in construction to frame activity and stimulate him. Include his family as much as possible and talk about them. Allow Jaheem to make as many decisions as possible – do not argue with him.	Put Jaheem in control of care situations. Don't force things on him; ask if he thinks it would be a good idea to do something and respect his decision. Use care as a way for Jaheem to show his abilities, and praise him without infantilising him. Be respectful of his age and position – this matters to Jaheem.

Chapter 8

Bridget – Pain

> Bridget is 82 years old and was diagnosed with dementia three years ago. She was admitted to hospital one week ago with a chest infection and swollen ankles. She has arthritis and takes regular medicine for this at home. Initially, she was suspicious of staff and refused to take medication and drinks. She tries to bite staff and punch them when they move her and shouts 'bear' repeatedly. Staff have transferred her to a side room because she was disturbing the other patients. In order to deliver care, the team has been giving her sedation, which has had little effect. Her oral intake is poor and she has lost four kilograms since being admitted. She scored 9/10 when assessed with a dementia-pain assessment tool. She has been given regular liquid analgesia and a patch for her arthritis. Today it is noted that her behaviour has reverted back to normal with no repetition, shouting or aggression and she has started to eat and drink again.

WHAT IS PAIN?

Pain is so universal that it is essential that it is recognised by all people working with older people; it places a blight on daily life, limiting functional ability and impairing the quality of life. The symptom manifests itself in many ways, not only as a sensory experience but also by causing psychological distress. (Philp 2007)

Pain is described as an unpleasant sensory and emotional experience associated with actual or potential damage to tissue – for example, a burn to the hand from an iron or a broken bone from a fall. Pain is always subjective – no other person can experience an individual's pain or know what it feels like or how it affects that person physically and emotionally.

Melzack and Casey (1968) identified the three dimensions of pain that have shaped current thinking (see Table 8.1). A person with dementia will experience difficulties with all these dimensions.

Table 8.1: Three dimensions of pain and how they impact on Bridget

Dimension	Meaning	How this can affect Bridget?
Sensory – discriminative	Sense of intensity and location, quality and duration.	Bridget might not be able to identify the location of her pain.
Affective – motivational	Unpleasantness and the urge to escape it.	Because Bridget is unable to explain what is happening, she is likely to express her urge to escape the pain as behaviour such as aggression or trying to leave.
Cognitive – evaluative	Appraisal, cultural values, meaning and distraction.	Bridget will not be able to understand the meaning of her pain or be able to distract herself from it.

PERCEPTION OF PAIN

Pain is a perception in the same way that vision and hearing are. This perception is real, whether or not harm has occurred or is occurring. Because of this, a person's emotional state and understanding of pain will have a significant effect on how it is experienced. Twycross and Lack (1983) identified key factors which affect pain tolerance, either increasing or decreasing it, and these are shown in Table 8.2.

Table 8.2: The key factors affecting pain tolerance

Aspects that lower tolerance	Aspects that raise tolerance
Insomnia	Relief of symptoms
Fatigue	Sleep
Anxiety	Rest or, paradoxically, physiotherapy
Fear	Relaxation therapy
Anger	Explanation/support
Sadness	Understanding/empathy
Depression	Diversional activity
Boredom	Companionship/listening
Mental isolation	Elevation of mood
Social abandonment	Understanding of the meaning and significance of pain
Introversion	Social inclusion
	Encouragement to express emotions

For Bridget, being in hospital and having dementia would both contribute to emotions identified in the first column, particularly fear, fatigue, isolation and boredom. These factors would exacerbate her pain experience.

PAIN IN A PERSON WITH DEMENTIA

Research has shown that pain in patients with dementia is often poorly recognised and under-treated. In one study, patients with dementia in hospital were 50 per cent less likely to receive analgesia than patients without dementia (Morrison and Siu 2000).

REASONS WHY PAIN IS POORLY MANAGED IN DEMENTIA PATIENTS

- As her disease progresses, Bridget may lose the ability to express herself verbally. The increasing pain will also affect her cognition and further reduce her ability to communicate.

- Myths exist that patients with dementia do not experience pain or, because memory is so poor, that they will forget it.

- Healthcare professionals often have poor knowledge of how to assess pain in patients who are non-verbal.

- Bridget's extreme behaviour will be attributed to her dementia and result in her being treated with psychotropic drugs rather than analgesia. No one will consider looking for a cause of her behaviour beyond having dementia.

COMMON CAUSES OF PAIN IN PEOPLE WITH DEMENTIA

Patients with dementia have a high probability of pain; dementia is most prevalent in older people and pain from conditions such as arthritis is common in this group. Like Bridget, patients often stop taking long-term medication when they are unwell or find themselves in an unfamiliar environment, and this can result in increased pain.

Other common causes of pain in patients with dementia are the simple ailments which afflict everyone, such as toothache and headache. When untreated, these can cause extreme distress, yet can be effectively managed with simple analgesia.

Staff need to be vigilant when older patients present with conditions such as constipation, urinary tract infections and pressure ulcers. Often, these conditions are not perceived as painful by clinicians, and patients who are unable to articulate pain miss out on being given analgesia. Pain is most often incidental or procedural – for example, when the person is being turned in bed or when a dressing is being cleaned or removed.

EXPRESSION OF PAIN IN DEMENTIA

Bridget is expressing pain through behaviour and this is common in people who have advanced dementia or communication difficulties. The person might struggle with conceptualisation of the pain and therefore be unable to identify the cause of the distress. There is strong evidence to show that there is a close correlation between extreme behaviours and the presence of pain in people with dementia (Husebo 2011 *et al.*; Lord *et al.* 2013). Common behaviours that would suggest pain are identified in Figure 8.1.

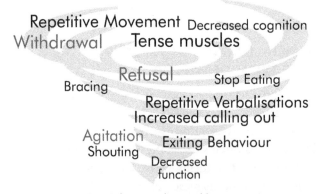

Repetitive Movement Decreased cognition
Withdrawal   Tense muscles

Refusal   Stop Eating
Bracing

Repetitive Verbalisations
Increased calling out

Agitation   Exiting Behaviour
Shouting
Decreased
function

Figure 8.1: Behaviours that would suggest pain

CORE PRINCIPLES OF PAIN ASSESSMENT

All older people should be asked about pain. Assessment should include both verbal and observational components. When verbally assessing for pain, the clinician must ensure that the right words are used to maximise understanding. Keep questions simple as some people may not understand the concept of 'pain'; it might be necessary to use words like 'sore' or 'does it hurt'. Remember that people with dementia might lose word recognition and therefore it might be necessary to try different words in questions. Research has shown that visual and numerical pain assessment tools have limited accuracy in patients with dementia (Lord *et al.* 2013) and therefore are not recommended.

OBSERVATIONAL PAIN ASSESSMENT

Behaviours potentially indicating the presence of pain vary enormously from individual to individual and can also vary in the same individual. Some patients may show very subtle changes. It should be remembered that such behaviours may have causes other than pain (see Chapter 11). All types of unusual behaviour should therefore be comprehensively monitored and their causes considered. To support observational assessment, the American Geriatrics Society (AGS) (2002) identified six observable components of pain:

- facial expression
- body movements
- verbalisations/vocalisations
- interpersonal reactions
- change in activity
- mental status changes.

These form the basis of the observation assessment tools which have been developed for people with dementia.

DEMENTIA-SPECIFIC PAIN ASSESSMENT TOOLS

There are numerous pain assessment tools available to identify pain in a person with dementia, and while these can be useful, it is important for the clinician to remember that the most important thing is to be aware of the possibility of pain. However, in Bridget's case, using a tool provided the evidence that there was pain and the means to monitor the effect of the analgesia she received. The City of Hope website (http://prc. coh.org/pain_assessment.asp) compares many of these tools and analyses them and is a useful resource when considering which one to use. All tools should be used in conjunction with history taking and a discussion with the carer/family member around a person's usual behaviour. Within the acute hospital setting, the two pain assessment tools commonly used are PAINAD (see Figure 8.2) and Abbey (see Figure 8.3). Both are effective and quick ways to assess pain.

Items	0	1	2	Score
Breathing independent of vocalisation	Normal	Occasional laboured breathing. Short period of hyperventilation.	Noisy, laboured breathing. Long period of hyperventilation. Cheyne-Stokes respirations.	
Negative vocalisation	None	Occasional moan or groan. Low-level speech with a negative or disapproving quality.	Repeated troubled calling out. Loud moaning or groaning. Crying.	
Facial expression	Smiling or inexpressive	Sad. Frightened. Frown.	Facial grimacing.	
Body language	Relaxed	Tense. Distressed pacing. Fidgeting.	Rigid. Fists clenched. Knees pulled up. Pulling or pushing away. Striking out.	
Consolability	No need to console	Distracted or reassured by voice or touch.	Unable to console, distract or reassure.	
			Total	

Figure 8.2: PAINAD (Warden, Hurley and Volicer 2003)

Abbey Pain Scale

For measurement of pain in people with dementia who cannot verbalise

How to use scale: while observing the resident score questions 1 to 6

Name of resident: _____

Name and designation of person completing the scale: _____

Date: _____ Time: _____

Latest pain relief given was: _____ at: _____ hrs

Q1 Vocalisation
e.g.whimpering, groaning, crying
Absent 0   Mild 1   Moderate 2   Severe 3

Q1 ☐

Q2 Facial expression
e.g. looking tense, frowning, grimacing, looking frightened
Absent 0   Mild 1   Moderate 2   Severe 3

Q2 ☐

Q3 Change in body language
e.g.fidgeting, rocking, guarding part of body, withdrawn
Absent 0   Mild 1   Moderate 2   Severe 3

Q3 ☐

Q4 Behavioural change
e.g. increased confusion, refusing to eat, alteration in usual patterns
Absent 0   Mild 1   Moderate 2   Severe 3

Q4 ☐

Q5 Physiological change
e.g. temperature, pulse of blood pressure outside normal limits, perspiring, flushing or pallor
Absent 0   Mild 1   Moderate 2   Severe 3

Q5 ☐

Q6 Physical changes
e.g. skin tears, pressure areas, arthritis, contractures, previous injuries
Absent 0   Mild 1   Moderate 2   Severe 3

Q6 ☐

Add scores for 1–6 and record here ⟶ Total pain score ☐

Now tick the box that matches the total pain score ⟶

0–2 No pain	3–7 Mild	8–13 Moderate	14+ Severe

Finally, tick the box which matches the type of pain ⟶

Chronic	Acute	Acute on chronic

Abbey, J., De Bellis, A., Piller, N., Easterman, A., Giles, L., Parker, D. and Lowcay, B.
Funded by JH and JD Gunn Medical Research Foundation 1998–2002.

Figure 8.3: Abbey Pain Scale (Abbey *et al.* 1998)

ADMINISTERING MEDICATION TO A PERSON WITH DEMENTIA

Bridget was refusing medication and this meant that she did not receive her regular analgesic. She was distrustful of the staff and also suspicious of the medicine pot. The staff response to this was to document that she had refused. However, simply documenting that the person will not take medication is not acceptable as the refusal might be intrinsically linked with the pain itself and therefore needs to be addressed.

The first consideration in this situation is what the best route of administration might be; for Bridget it was a combination of liquid analgesia and a patch. There is often more success when using non-tablet forms of analgesia with people who have dementia, as tablets often have negative connotations and might be difficult to swallow.

NON-PHARMACOLOGICAL METHODS TO ALLEVIATE PAIN

Pain can be exacerbated in hospital for a person with dementia because of factors such as boredom and loneliness. Clinicians should also seek non-pharmacological means to support the patient and reduce pain:

- Gentle exercises to relieve stiff joints (seek advice from a physiotherapist).

- Aromatherapy to reduce tension in muscles.

- Gentle massage to relieve tight muscles.

- Heat pads – caution should be used so that they do not irritate and are not too hot or used for too long.

- Positioning the person so that they are comfortable in bed or in a chair.

- Use of air mattress and air cushions to alleviate pressure.

- Distraction, relieving boredom, calm, comfortable environment, social contact, treating anxiety and/or depression can all help to alleviate pain.

How to make best practice happen

Have I asked why Bridget is reacting this way?	Bridget does not normally behave this way. Do a pain assessment and also look for the source of her pain. What happens when she is given pain relief?	
What are Bridget's strengths/ abilities?	Bridget is able to communicate verbally and physically through her behaviour. Bridget has always been strong and coped well with problems.	
	Qualified staff	**Healthcare support worker**
Am I listening?	If you listen to the emotion in her voice rather than the words she is using, you can hear that Bridget is distressed. Her voice is strained and she sounds unhappy. Perseveration (repeating the same word over and over) is a recognised pain-related behaviour in a person with dementia.	Does Bridget sound happy? When does she become combative? She has history of arthritis and hits out when staff are moving her – what do her actions tell you?
Do I know enough about Bridget?	Bridget brought up four children and worked as a dinner lady at a school. Her daughter says that she was very tough and did not like to make a fuss about being ill or in pain; she would keep herself busy to take her mind off it. Keep Bridget busy, as her pain will be more manageable if she is distracted. You can use her interest in food to distract her and encourage her to eat and drink.	Discuss Bridget's past hobbies and likes with her and her family. Use the information to engage with Bridget and keep her mind stimulated and busy.

	Qualified staff	**Healthcare support worker**
What can I do to enable Bridget?	Use Bridget's ability to communicate to gauge how she is. Use a pain assessment tool to observe Bridget and score her pain. When she was given analgesia, Bridget stopped shouting and fighting, and therefore this can be used as a measure of her level of discomfort.	Always respond to her behaviour by asking, 'What is Bridget telling me?' Involve Bridget in food and drink as this will be familiar to her. Engage her in conversation about her children and her past hobbies. Bridget likes to keep herself busy, so ensure that she is never left unstimulated.

Chapter 9

Myrtle – Eating and Drinking

Myrtle is 90 years old, has a diagnosis of dementia and lives in a residential home. She was admitted to hospital after a fall from a chair and has been drowsy, uncommunicative and disengaged on the ward. She has not made any attempt to eat or drink independently so staff are attempting to assist her. This results in Myrtle becoming agitated and combative, going for long periods throughout the day without any oral intake. Doctors have begun treating Myrtle for a urinary tract infection (UTI) and have prescribed regular analgesia.

It has also been identified that Myrtle has a hypoactive delirium. Staff are worried that she will deteriorate due to her lack of oral intake and have therefore tried to gain information from Myrtle's residential home regarding strategies on how they can support her.

Food and drink provide our bodies with nutrients that are essential for growth, good health and survival. A lack of appetite is common in the elderly as well as the partial or total loss of senses important for nutrition, such as taste and smell.

A diagnosis of dementia might lead to alterations in a person's ability to independently manage their own nutrition and hydration; this results in problems with managing all aspects of eating and drinking. In the hospital setting, eating and drinking often take a back seat to the medical needs of the patient and so the risk of malnutrition and dehydration can increase. A recent study stated that 70 per cent of elderly patients in hospital suffer from malnutrition (Guerchet *et al.* 2014).

IMPORTANCE OF ADEQUATE NUTRITION AND HYDRATION IN HOSPITAL

Nutrition

Nutrients are involved in health and recovery in a variety of ways, and if a patient has poor oral intake, their body and health can suffer due to a lack of these. During an acute admission, it is vital that the body gets the nutrients it needs to maintain and repair internal organs and tissues that may have been damaged. Inadequate nutrition results in additional morbidities, delays in discharge and even mortality (Archibald 2006).

Myrtle's hypoactive delirium and cognitive impairment led to a poor intake of food and fluid from the beginning of her admission. This put her at risk of malnutrition, weight loss, elongated recovery time, low energy levels and constipation.

To assess risk of malnutrition, patients will have a nutrition assessment completed by nursing staff on admission and regularly throughout their stay. All hospitals will have a specific tool to assess each patient's nutritional status and whether they are malnourished or at risk of becoming malnourished. This assessment will consider factors such as the patient's age, their body mass index (BMI), any recent weight loss and any acute illnesses. If the patient is considered to be malnourished, or at risk, based on this assessment, a referral to a dietician should be completed in order for them to support the patient with specialist dietary support and advice.

Hydration

Many elderly patients get admitted to hospital with dehydration or develop it during their stay. Similar to nutrition, people with dementia may struggle to keep themselves sufficiently hydrated while in hospital. Figure 9.1 shows how water is utilised by the body.

Myrtle was dehydrated, had a urinary tract infection and was constipated when she was admitted. It is thought that she stopped drinking and developed the urinary tract infection and constipation as a result of this. She subsequently became so unwell that she lost interest in drinking and this further exacerbated the problem. Her case illustrates the snowball effect that poor hydration can have with an older person.

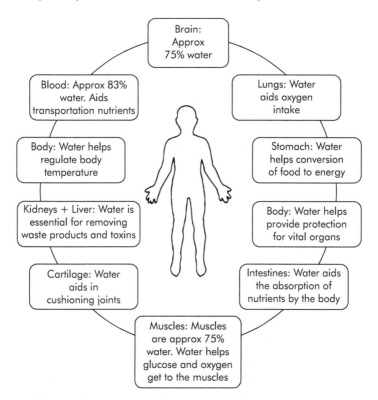

Figure 9.1: The importance of water to support function (Kendall 2015)

COMMON PROBLEMS

As a person's dementia progresses, they are likely to experience difficulties with eating and drinking. Common problems include:

- forgetting that they have eaten or thinking that they have eaten when they have not

- choosing foods or remembering how to prepare food

- being unable to open food packaging

- getting the food to their mouth

- remembering to chew and swallow the food when it is in their mouth

- problems with eating harder foods due to dental problems

- problems recognising foods and distinguishing between edible and non-edible items

- changing of tastes – people with dementia will often prefer sweeter or spicier foods

- forgetting how to use cutlery or recognising the cutlery

- forgetting how to get a cup/glass to their mouth or not recognising the cup/glass

- development of swallowing problems as the disease progresses

- loss of appetite.

REDUCED ORAL INTAKE IN HOSPITAL

Like Myrtle, many people with dementia experience increased cognitive and functional impairment when they are in hospital and this can exacerbate problems with eating and drinking. Table 9.1 details the issues associated with cognitive, physical and environmental factors that can lead to reduced oral intake for a patient with dementia during a hospital stay.

Table 9.1: Problems associated with poor intake in people with dementia

Cognitive	Physical	Environmental
Problems recognising/ coordinating food, cutlery, crockery.	Trouble bringing cutlery or cup to the mouth.	Unfamiliar surroundings.
Struggling to get food or drink to their mouth.	Ill-fitting dentures.	Environment being too hot and too dry.
Orientation to time – e.g. thinking it's night time when food is being served.	Pain – reducing appetite, reducing ability to sit up/chew/ swallow.	Being in bed for long periods – reducing appetite, increasing drowsiness.
Orientation to place – e.g. thinking they are in a restaurant and having no money to pay.	Problems visualising food, cutlery, dishes, cups and so on due to eyesight problems.	Bad lighting. Loud, busy ward. Rushed mealtimes.
Unable to verbalise a dislike regarding food/drink.	Problems ordering food due to expressive or auditory difficulties.	Having to wait to be assisted.
Delirium or agitation reducing ability to engage at mealtimes.		Spending mealtimes alone.
Remembering to swallow/holding food in the mouth.		

STRATEGIES TO ENCOURAGE EATING AND DRINKING

Cater for the patient's preferences

After discovering a person's likes and dislikes it is important to ensure that they actually receive food and drink that they like. Reeling off a list of options from a menu may confuse a patient who will struggle to order something they like, commonly ordering the last thing that was heard. Additionally, patients with dementia may not be able to voice dissatisfaction with food they receive. A person's tastes can change with dementia and so previous likes and dislikes may not be current ones.

Things to do:

- Listen to the patient, family members and care givers regarding the patient's usual likes/dislikes.

- Use pictorial menus when ordering food with patients to help them visualise what they are ordering.

- If a patient with dementia says they do not like something that you have been told they do like, cater for what the person is telling you – tastes may have changed.

Like many older people, Myrtle saw water as something for washing in rather than drinking and refused to drink the water in hospital. It was a simple thing that was not discovered for a few days and resulted in further dehydration. After this, staff began providing fruit squash instead of the usual jug of water and the improvement in Myrtle's fluid intake was remarkable.

Identifying pain

Pain is commonly unrecognised in people with dementia and they will not always express any pain they are experiencing (see Chapter 7); this can have a detrimental effect on appetite and intake. If someone is in pain, that person is less likely to engage at mealtimes and may not be able to sit up to eat and drink.

Things to do:

- Regularly assess pain using an assessment tool specific for people with dementia.

Myrtle had been admitted after a fall and a broken hip was suspected. She was experiencing significant levels of pain in areas affected by the fall and was often uncomfortable at mealtimes when she was sitting out of bed. The medical team prescribed regular analgesia, which helped manage Myrtle's pain and enabled her to enjoy her meals.

Positioning

In hospitals, patients are often left to eat meals while lying in bed at awkward angles or in a semi-prone position. Patients with dementia may struggle with eating in bed for several reasons:

- discomfort due to bad positioning
- aspirating food because of not sitting up straight
- thinking it is night time and not normal to have a meal
- difficulty managing to get the food from plate to mouth when reclining.

Things to do:

- Transfer the patient out of bed to a chair at mealtimes.
- Sit the patient upright in bed with the table across them if they are unable to transfer to a chair.
- Orientate the person to time regularly so that they know mealtimes are approaching.

While in bed, Myrtle was very drowsy and struggled to eat or drink. When out of bed, she was much more alert and her intake increased. It was therefore ensured that Myrtle was transferred out of bed every day, especially for mealtimes, and this made her more alert and willing to eat and drink.

Identifying depression

People experiencing depression will commonly have reduced oral intake. Depression can cause a person to become introverted, quiet and less likely to engage; these are all behaviours which a person with dementia might exhibit. Due to this similarity, depression is often missed in people with dementia as these symptoms are frequently attributed to progressing dementia.

Things to do:

- Complete an assessment for depression such as the Geriatric Depression Scale (GDS) or the Hospital Anxiety and Depression Scale (HADS).

- Look for a history of depression.

- Look for signs of depression.

- Notify the medical team of any depressive characteristics.

In Myrtle's case, it was identified that she had developed depression while at the residential home and this was part of the reason for her lack of interest in food and drink. Anti-depressants were prescribed and following this Myrtle became more alert, looked brighter and would smile at staff when they were talking to her. Additionally, her appetite came back and her intake began to increase.

Social eating

Eating and drinking are social acts. Friends often get together over drinks or a meal and families will eat their meals sitting around a table. Yet, in hospital, patients are mostly left to eat in isolation with little human contact. Sitting around a table on the ward with other patients can give the meal a more social feel and be a more familiar way of eating.

Things to do:

- Have group meals where patients sit around a table to eat.

- Organise social events such as tea parties on the ward.

- Sit with a patient at mealtimes and speak with them, keeping conversation relative to the meal.

- Join patients with your own lunch.

Staff started to spend time with Myrtle at mealtimes and also involved her in ward tea parties at which members of staff were amazed at how much Myrtle would eat.

Music at mealtimes

Music is known to reduce agitation and lift mood in patients with dementia. Discovering certain musical preferences will enable you to provide music that the patient will be familiar with and may elicit fond memories of their past.

Things to do:

• Discover what music a person likes.

• Provide CD players or radios and play music throughout the day and during meals.

Myrtle was provided with familiar music that was played during meals; this lifted her mood and she was often seen swaying and humming to the music.

Knowing when to assist

Myrtle's delirium and dementia stopped her from initiating anything, which meant that she would simply turn away or not move when food was served. The ward staff assumed that she needed assistance, but when they tried to feed her, she would become distressed and push them away. Once it was discovered that Myrtle could eat independently with the right encouragement, environment and guidance, nursing staff were able to help Myrtle to feed herself.

Promoting the independence of patients is imperative while they are in hospital. Patients with dementia can lose functional ability around eating and drinking (such as remembering how to feed themselves) when they are given too much assistance. Therefore, the aim should always be to maximise independence by getting the patient to eat and drink independently, but this takes time and encouragement. If a patient requires help initiating the task, you can try:

- reminding them the food is there

- handing them the cutlery

- describing the food to them

- putting food onto the cutlery for them.

These little steps of assistance often lead to the person maintaining independence. Of course, if a patient does require full assistance, then it is important that they receive it; however, staff should go at their pace and not let other pressures interfere with this social act that should be made enjoyable for that person.

The reasons why a person like Myrtle will stop eating and drinking in hospital are multifactorial and intrinsically linked to culture, taste, mood and physical well-being. Clinicians need to understand the value of maintaining good hydration and nutrition in people with dementia, but also appreciate the complex nature of a refusal and how it can be addressed.

How to make best practice happen

Have I asked why Myrtle is reacting this way?	Myrtle's delirium, depression and pain are hampering her ability to eat and drink.
	Treating these will be the first step.
	Myrtle is delirious and depressed and therefore does not want to eat.
	Myrtle does not like being fed and will refuse to eat if you try to feed her.
	Myrtle does not like water and will not drink it if it is offered to her.
What are Myrtle's strengths/ abilities?	Myrtle can feed herself more effectively with her hands and she can hold a cup.
	Myrtle has good social skills and enjoys engaging with other people.

	Qualified staff	Healthcare support worker
Am I listening?	Myrtle's agitation is a form of communication and staff must look for the reasons behind it. Myrtle's agitation on being assisted to eat and drink is because she likes to do things for herself and doesn't like being helped.	If Myrtle becomes agitated, understand that it is her way of communicating and not simply her dementia. Find ways to support Myrtle that don't lead to her becoming agitated and ensure that they are implemented on your shifts.
Do I know enough about Myrtle?	Investigate Myrtle's usual eating and drinking habits. Myrtle is a very independent lady and has always done things for herself. Ensure that Myrtle is sat out of bed for meals and allowed to eat and drink independently with verbal encouragement.	Sit with Myrtle and give her verbal encouragement to eat – do not feed her.
What can I do to enable Myrtle?	Provide finger foods as much as possible and enable her to eat meals without physical assistance. Use Myrtle's social nature to help engage her in social events such as tea parties or even simply sitting her with other patients at mealtimes.	Ensure that Myrtle can reach her cup and that it is always filled with something she likes to drink. Make sure any finger foods that are available are within easy reach and remind Myrtle that they are there regularly. Talk to Myrtle throughout the day to give that sense of being social. Ensure that Myrtle can reach her food and do not try to assist her if you think she is going too slowly.

Chapter 10

Geoffrey – Getting Someone to Move (Enabling, Goal Setting and Engaging)

Geoffrey has been admitted to the acute medical unit (AMU) after sustaining a fall at home, a laceration to his right eye and a painful right wrist. He had been found this morning by his carer who had seen him last night and noticed that Geoffrey 'wasn't his usual self'. On AMU, it is noted that Geoffrey is 'restless' and continues to try and get out of bed. Investigations showed his urine dip to be positive for proteins and leucocytes, and he has therefore been started on a course of antibiotics. An x-ray of his right wrist shows a colles fracture and a plastercast has been applied.

As Geoffrey has not yet been seen by the physiotherapist or occupational therapist, the nursing staff have kept him in bed to reduce the risk of him falling on the ward. Geoffrey has become withdrawn and declines to engage with medical or nursing interventions on the ward. He is being transferred to the surgical rehabilitation unit for ongoing input.

INTRODUCTION

Promoting and maintaining mobility is an essential aspect of caring for people with dementia (Jootun and Pryde 2013). As dementia progresses, it can affect the parts of the brain that are responsible for maintaining one's balance and ability to control movement patterns. Individuals with dementia can often misunderstand their physical environment, resulting in complications with deciding what sights and sounds are most important to them. After an acute illness such as a urine infection or a chest infection, specialist therapy input is not necessarily indicated, as encouragement and practice alone will usually help individuals back onto their feet. However, there are many intrinsic and extrinsic challenges staff face when moving and handling people with dementia. This chapter aims to offer guidance on how to deal with these challenges, to promote safe practice and improve patient outcomes.

WHAT ARE THE DIFFICULTIES STAFF COME UP AGAINST?

There are many difficulties staff can face when helping someone with dementia to move; however, there is no single intervention known to be particularly effective and other factors must be considered. The safe handling of patients with dementia is never without risk to the handler but there appears to be limited guidance on how to handle patients with cognitive impairments (Wright 2005). It is vital to understand the task in hand, the environment the patient is in – bedside, toilet, armchair and so on – and the individual personal factors.

Difficulties with mobility can occur more often in some types of dementia than in others. For example, rigid movement patterns are characteristic of fronto-temporal dementia, Lewy Body, Parkinson's disease dementia, and a group of dementias associated with so-called 'Parkinson-plus' disorders.

Associated medical conditions such as arthritis, gout and cancer can also make movements painful, which will reduce an individual's ability to engage in mobility and activities of daily living and also play havoc with an individual's confidence.

Mobility
To be able to move about either on your own or with the use of a walking aid.

The loss of mobility associated with damaged areas in the brain can lead to even more physical complaints as well as contributing to depression and social isolation.

The non-use and misuse of mobility aids and assistive technology is also a concern. Staff should only use mobility aids with patients who are able to comprehend the purpose of them; otherwise they can end up being a tripping hazard. There are many ways in which staff can use an individual's behaviours to support mobility levels on a ward.

Staff members must consider the following steps:

- Understand how dementia affects mobility.

- Know the techniques involved in safe handling.

- Understand the necessity for accurate risk assessment.

- Know the significance of the patient's premorbid mobility level and the current 'advised' level of assistance (not too much/not too little).

The ultimate goal is 'the equipping of individuals to live in ways that they have previously enjoyed, with or without the assistance of others' (Dewing 2003). With regard to Geoffrey, he was a man living at home, relatively independent, with a care package supporting him with his morning and evening wash. He mobilised independently unaided, and if staff had encouraged him to move rather than disable him, he might have been discharged home from the AMU, which would have reduced his length of stay.

WHAT AFFECTS A PERSON'S MOBILITY?

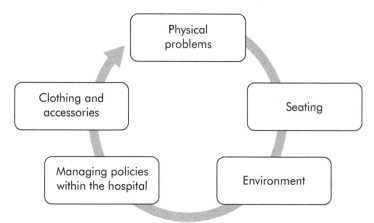

Figure 10.1: What affects a person's mobility?

Figure 10.1 shows the different ways in which a person's mobility can be affected in hospital. Dementia can have a major impact on the individual's ability to make sense of their environment. Individuals can experience a slowing down of responses and actions (Killick and Allan 2001). McKeefry and Bartlett (2010) found that people with dementia can have reduced visual acuity, contrast sensitivity, colour vision, spatial awareness and depth perception. The ability of a person to cope with visual impairment can influence their cognitive performance and their ability to mobilise and engage in activities of daily living.

Clinicians need to be aware that sometimes a person's freedom of movement can be restricted unintentionally while in hospital. Examples of this are shown below:

- *Physical complications.* Mobility may be reduced by a simple lack of thought about the person's physical environment. Providing a chair which is too low or too high for an individual to get out of, leaving a person on a commode or in a chair for too long or tucking in bed clothes too tight for a person who tends to walk about at night are all factors that may have an effect on reducing someone's ability to mobilise. It is also important to remember that people with dementia can have problems with walking that are not due to the dementia itself. Fatigue and pain can limit how far a person can walk. Sometimes pain can reflect an unattended problem in foot care.

- *Medication.* Too many drugs can lead to a loss of mobility, which can further result in muscle shortening/ contractures. Patients with dementia must only be given medication that is in their best interests, and sedatives are best avoided unless they are prescribed to address specific medical difficulties.

WHAT DO YOU DO TO OVERCOME THESE DIFFICULTIES?

Remington *et al.* (2006) acknowledged that no single intervention can be universally effective in ameliorating behaviour and that individualised ones are the most effective.

- *Sound.* Engage with your patient through the use of a calm and reassuring tone of voice, clear, short sentences, saying the patient's name, building a rapport with the patient and giving positive instructions. The most effective communication tool is offering simple and clear step-by-step instructions followed by repeated verbal cues and prompts (Varnam 2011).

- *Physical.* Sander (2002) outlined how staff members can guide the movements of a patient with their own body movements. Dance is also known to be used as a means of initiating movement, and as a distraction to produce a positive behaviour from a negative one.

- *Visual.* Visual responses such as mime, gestures and good eye contact are all of utmost importance when an individual is struggling to process a verbal instruction.

- *Equipment and environment.* Floor surfaces are environmental factors which staff members have no control over, but a verbal prompt and reassurance can sometimes relieve the patient of any sensory discomfort or environmental misunderstanding – for example, reassuring the patient that the floor is shiny rather than wet. Always ensure that the environment is free of clutter and loud background noises.

Varnam (2011) found that sound and physical interventions had the best success rates in a study conducted looking at the sit-to-stand transfer. Carefully constructed and repeated instructions communicated in a reassuring manner, with tactile stimulation to guide movement, are known to have the greater success rate when mobilising patients. Sander (2002) confirms this by highlighting the efficacy of appropriate nods and smiles, and noted that signs of irritability from the caregiver can make the person with dementia anxious. Spending time with your patients is hugely beneficial but the ward environment and complex caseloads that staff members manage can prevent this. Ward routines can be time-consuming and prevent this quality patient contact (Gustafsson and Fagerberg 2004). A decline in an individual's functional ability can result in 'doing for' rather than 'doing with'. This highlights the importance of finding out about your patient (baseline level of function), setting the patient up for the task, standing back and intervening only when you observe a patient struggle or ask for help.

There are types of problems with starting to walk (with gait ignition disorders) that respond to a variety of actions known as 'sensory tricks': for example, vigorously stroking the leg that you want the person to start moving, or seeing if they can lift their feet up and down to march on the spot, or seeing if they can step over something to start – such as a line. As Geoffrey had spent years in the armed services he responded very well to the command 'quick march' when spoken softly into his ear.

Other behaviours to support an individual's ability to mobilise include the following:

- Use the information provided by the patient, their carers and other professionals to ensure that you are clear in your expectations about how much you will need to do, what equipment you'll need and how much assistance the patient will need.

- Explain the task and its purpose to the patient.

- Ask the patient to do as much as they can themselves and give them time to respond.

- Repeat the explanation as frequently as required.

- Place the appropriate walking aid in position and ensure that the patient understands what it is.

- Ask the patient to put on their slippers/shoes or assist them with this task and ensure that they are fitting correctly.

- Move furniture that is intruding the space – for example, bedside tables.

- Good moving and handling techniques involve thinking before moving. Plan what the task is that you want to achieve with the patient and how you are going to achieve it.

- Prior to starting to mobilise, adopt a stable position next to your patient.

- Start moving and handling the patient with a good posture, making sure that you bend your back, hips and knees slightly. Do not stoop or fully flex your knees and hips.

Effective communication is imperative when you are encouraging someone with dementia to mobilise. Worsening of dual-task performance/multi-tasking (doing two things at once, such as talking while walking) is often associated with competing demands for attentional resources. In other words, patients with dementia are unable to divert their attention to two different tasks at the same time.

- *Processing the information.* Processing information will take an individual longer than it used to, so be patient. If you try to hurry them, they may feel under pressure. Ask how they are, wait for an answer, and perhaps repeat the question.

- *Understanding.* Many people with dementia find it difficult to understand what they are being asked to do. It is up to you to ensure that the patient comprehends by making use of the approaches and cues previously discussed.

- *Memory.* When memory loss embeds itself, people find it difficult to remember what they have been asked to do, or what they are doing currently. In this case, you may need to repeat your instruction several times; use key words or physically demonstrate the step of the task to help the individual complete the task.

- *Expressing themselves.* When a person with dementia is verbally or non-verbally communicating that they do not want to do something, we need to understand why. It might be how the person is interpreting the situation – for example, they may feel as if they are being talked down to and are refusing in order to keep a sense of control. Ensure that you talk to the patient, be honest about their progress, listen to their wishes and work in partnership with them.

- *Your communication.* Use repetition generously, speak clearly with simple instructions and give the person enough time to respond. Consider all sensory impairments – if the patient has a hearing impairment, write instructions down or use physical gesture/demonstrations, and so on.

How to make best practice happen

Have I asked why Geoffrey is reacting this way?	When Geoffrey is trying to get out of bed we should assist him with this rather than confine him to his bed. Geoffrey has a new fracture and is obviously going to be in pain; do you think Geoffrey is having enough pain relief?
	Why is Geoffrey trying to climb out of bed?
	Does he need the toilet?
	Is he uncomfortable while lying down?

What are Geoffrey's strengths/abilities?	Geoffrey has always been physically active and we need to maintain this level of independence.
	Geoffrey spent years in the army and he responds well to the command 'quick march' when spoken softly to him.
	Use this physical ability to engage him in activities, as well as promoting independence in walking to the bathroom to wash and go to the toilet.

	Qualified staff	Healthcare support worker
Am I listening?	Have we listened to where Geoffrey has said he wants to go? Have we assessed for pain? Have we responded to Geoffrey's questions about his family?	What does Geoffrey want to do? Is there any reason why he cannot walk around if he wants to?
Do I know enough about Geoffrey?	Ask Geoffrey how he managed at home and if he has a carer. Was he able to walk unaided? Unless you know otherwise, assume that there are no issues with his mobility and get him out of bed within the first few hours of his admission, provided that he is medically well.	Make sure you know Geoffrey's past hobbies and career as well as his mobility baseline. Ask the physio team to assess him so you can safely support him with mobilising around the ward. Geoffrey's time in the armed services means he responds well to concise commands such as 'quick march'.

What can I do to enable Geoffrey?	Ensure that Geoffrey understands what you are asking him to do. Complete a pain assessment tool to ensure that Geoffrey is not in pain.	Keep commands short and simple, do not give too many commands at once, and leave time for a response from Geoffrey.
	Ensure that are fully aware of his baseline level of mobility and hand this information over to all appropriate members of the multidisciplinary team.	Explain the task clearly to Geoffrey and why you are doing it, giving him time to process the information.
	Ensure that Geoffrey has access to the right mobility aid if he needs one and provide him with a suitable armchair.	Ensure that the environment is ready for the task before you proceed so you can concentrate on Geoffrey during it.

Chapter 11

Kenny – Different Behaviour

Kenny was admitted to hospital with severe abdominal pain, aggression and confusion. He has a known history of dementia. The abdominal pain has resolved with paracetamol but Kenny remains aggressive towards staff.

Kenny is described as 'confused', 'a wanderer', 'difficult', 'violent' and 'verbally and physically aggressive'. He has left the ward on two occasions and was brought back by staff. The ward manager confronted Kenny and he reacted aggressively by punching her in the face. There are strong concerns over his behaviour and ability to care for himself independently at home. Kenny has been assessed as requiring one-to-one supervision while in hospital and has often shouted at the person observing him.

Staff find it increasingly difficult to communicate with Kenny as he struggles to understand what is being said, follow instructions and verbally express his needs and feelings. This situation is disturbing not only for Kenny but also for staff who are struggling to provide the care he requires.

WHY THE CHALLENGE?

Dementia is an obstruction to understanding the person. Once someone is diagnosed, it is too easy to ascribe any challenging behaviour to their dementia.

Unfortunately, Kenny is not alone in being labelled as having challenging behaviour. Ninety per cent of people with dementia will experience behaviours that we find challenging (Alzheimer's Society 2013) but it does not mean that the behaviours are caused by dementia. There are a number of different behaviours that we can find challenging which include hallucinations, depression, physical or verbal aggression, crying and repetitive behaviours (both verbal and physical). Dementia can cause changes to a person's behaviour and personality but, as with all of us, people with dementia are commonly affected by a variety of interactions between cognitive health, environmental factors, their physical health and how other people act towards them.

While in hospital, our patients have many of these factors impacting on them as well as their diagnosis of dementia, so it is easy to see why we come across different behaviours. A new environment, new faces and names, beeping machines and pagers, often a lack of natural light, and the person's physical illness and pain will all impact on their behaviour.

UNMET NEEDS

Cohen-Mansfield (2000) suggested that challenging behaviour in dementia often reflects an attempt by the person to signal that a need is currently not being met (for example, to indicate pain, boredom or being tired), or an effort by the individual to get their needs met directly (wanting to leave hospital to go to work), or as a sign of frustration (being blocked from leaving the ward they are on).

The unmet needs model proposes that challenging behaviours are created from a complex interaction between cognitive impairment, physical health, mental health, past habits, personality and environmental (physical and social) factors.

The unmet needs model provides a basis for assessing and understanding the potential causes of challenging behaviour instead of just focusing on the behaviour itself.

At the centre of this model is not just knowing the person, but also knowing ourselves and understanding why we all react in challenging ways.

With Kenny, there was no attempt at understanding why he was behaving this way, just an acceptance that he was. The ward staff maintained his safety by stopping him leaving the ward and placing him on one-to-one observations, but that actually made the situation worse for him and the staff. If the staff had thought of the unmet needs model, they could have approached it differently.

Kenny was a doorman at a club before he stopped working due to his dementia. During his working life, he dealt with aggressive and drunken people and had to defend himself on several occasions. His attempts to leave the ward were explained by his family; at home Kenny will often stand outside the front door of his flat. They believe that this is Kenny acting out his work as a doorman and the family have found no problems with letting him do this.

It is useful to look at four categories to try to find the reasons behind a person's behaviour.

HEALTH AND SENSORY CHANGES

Research conducted by Norway Care Homes (Husebo *et al.* 2011) and unpublished research from the BEPAID study (Lord *et al.* 2013) showed that there is a strong link between challenging behaviour and untreated pain (see Chapter 8). Other factors that can cause changes in behaviour include hunger, needing the toilet, lack of sleep and any primary illness. Sensory deficits will also contribute; if the patient is not wearing their hearing aid or glasses, then this will significantly impact on how they communicate, what they understand and how they react. Health and sensory changes can make the difference, with a patient not wanting to get out of bed, stopping eating and drinking, lashing out when staff try to give personal care and not engaging well with care. It is important that these aspects are considered when there are any changes in behaviour.

A diagnosis of dementia can change the way a person behaves too; if there are changes to the frontal lobe, they may have personality changes, become aggressive or have ritualistic behaviours. Dementia can also change how a person communicates; Kenny had a diagnosis of dementia with a progressive aphasic disorder which causes both receptive and expressive dysphasia (language impairment). He was unable to verbally express his needs and so when he was frightened, challenged or startled he would react through his behaviour.

OTHER PEOPLE

The way we act and talk and how fast we are going will impact on a person with dementia. The pace in hospital is usually fast; we have set tasks and limited time to achieve them. Unfortunately, this can cause a sensory overload in a person with dementia. In many situations the triggers for challenging behaviours can be linked to the carer being too rushed, abrupt and not empathetic (James 2011). This is an important factor to note as many instances of challenging behaviour occur during practical face-to-face interactions with the carer and patient. Good communication skills, 'going slow' and breaking tasks down into step-by-step instructions are important here. Give your full attention to the patient and keep the language and terms used simple.

Kenny reacted aggressively towards the staff because he felt threatened. Often, we stop patients from going somewhere in hospital because we want to keep them safe and on the ward, but we often block people with our bodies and use harsh words like 'stop', 'no' or 'don't go in there' which come across as aggressive. We can all think of a time when we felt threatened by someone else – we act differently in these situations and one way is aggressively. Kenny would talk about 'the man following me', referring to the member of staff on one-to-one observations with him. This role is often viewed as a punishment by patients: someone to guard them and stop them from doing things; one-to-one observation should be a positive interaction – an opportunity to get to know the patient and create a calming and social environment with entertainment and stimulation.

ENVIRONMENT

Environmental factors such as light, noise and layout are important influences on the well-being of many people, depending on their level of dependency. This is particularly the case for people with dementia who have difficulties with memory, problem solving and orientation. The environment can often be a barrier to engaging in fulfilling relationships (James 2011). It is important to check whether a patient's challenging behaviour might be triggered by them being too hot/cold, exposed to excess stimulation such as a loud television or radio, or a lack of signs telling them where they are (Dementia Services Development Centre 2008). Cunningham (2006) noted that aspects of the environment and care practice can lead to problems for the person with dementia, which may then be misinterpreted and lead to challenging behaviour. These included the stress of hospitalisation, transfer trauma (for example, when being transferred from A&E to the ward), being around unfamiliar people and in an unfamiliar environment. The Alzheimer's Society's *Counting the Cost* report (2009) found that just by an individual with dementia being in the hospital environment, their carers noticed a worsening of dementia symptoms and an increase in behavioural and psychological symptoms. A positive for Kenny was the fact that he was very mobile, so he was much more likely to familiarise himself with his environment on the ward.

LIFE HISTORY

How a person has lived their life will impact on how they behave when they have dementia. It is important also to recognise that a person's personality endures through the course of dementia and their individuality will be apparent in various ways and at different stages of their illness (James 2011). Knowing a person's preferences and normal routines can help to avoid challenging behaviours occurring at all; considering religious practices, dietary choices and coping mechanisms (for example, when stressed, the patient may like to go for a walk) are important in helping to make the time in hospital more consistent with their time at home as well as helping with challenging behaviour. Using a passport or personalised plan, such as the Alzheimer's Society leaflet 'This is Me', can provide staff with this type of information.

Knowing Kenny's history helped the staff understand what he was going through. The staff stopped blocking Kenny from leaving the ward and instead let him stand at the ward doors and took him out a cup of tea every now and then. This was a strategy that was agreed with the staff and his family and the aggression stopped.

WONDERING ABOUT THE WANDERER?

This is a behaviour that is constantly identified as challenging in hospitals but there are many reasons why people (not just with dementia!) walk. There are questions that we should ask inwardly when we find ourselves presented with 'wandering':

- Do you walk around every day?

- When you are at home, do you 'potter about'?

- Do you ever walk around or fidget when you are worried?

- Have you ever found that moving around can help when you are in pain?

We stop people from walking in hospital often as a protective measure as we do not want them to fall down or leave the ward and get lost, but, again, if we look at the person behind the behaviours, then we can understand their needs. Kenny was described as a wanderer, but walking around and standing at the main doors was part of his job; this was his normal routine, but as it did not fit into the idea of what a patient does in hospital, it became a challenging behaviour.

When we are faced with 'wandering', we need to think of it as purposeful; no one walks for no reason, so try to identify what the need is, meet it and it ceases to be a challenging behaviour.

Often the patient that we worry about the most is the 'falls risk' wanderer. It is important that these patients are still encouraged to walk, as without this exercise the risk of falls increases. Assess the amount of risk for Kenny, ascertaining whether he understands the risks of falling and whether he has capacity to make a decision about this (see Chapter 4).

Make a referral as soon as possible for a physiotherapist to review mobility. They will also be able to suggest interventions to help the person mobilise safely.

NON-PHARMACOLOGICAL INTERVENTIONS

There are many interventions that we can use to help calm, distract or occupy a person – anything as simple as a newspaper, a crossword, listening to the radio, dancing, a hand massage or a bit of gardening. Staff should be guided by the person's abilities and interests as well as available activities.

Non-pharmacological interventions should not be reactive or 'one-offs' or prescribed; they should not be checklists of activities for all patients. We should endeavour to find the person underneath the symptoms and the reasons behind the perceived challenging behaviours.

When we look at Kenny's situation on the ward, we can see that he kept trying to go out of the main doors; the ward staff saw this as a challenging and unsafe action and reacted by stopping him. They tried to distract him with newspapers, cups of tea and listening to music, but would often just block him, but Kenny found this to be an aggressive behaviour towards him and would respond equally with aggression. If the staff had spoken to his family, they would have discovered Kenny's profession and realised that since retirement and developing dementia he stands at his front door as if he is at work.

Allowing Kenny to carry out his routine also improved his verbal communication; Kenny would speak to staff, patients and visitors as he stood at the door or when he walked around the ward. He seemed much calmer and happier. He sometimes joked with staff, which his family stated was much more fitting with his personality. During his working life, Kenny would often do odd jobs around the club such as moving heavy boxes and equipment and DIY. This information can also be used to develop interventions such as moving boxes on the ward or asking advice about a piece of DIY. Kenny's sense of identity is then preserved and fulfilled.

There is not a one-size-fits-all approach to interventions in dementia. If we had asked Kenny to sit down for a hand massage or paint a picture, then this would not have met his underlying need for wanting to work as a doorman.

DE-ESCALATION TECHNIQUES

There may be times when a person with dementia becomes aggressive, causing a possible danger to themselves or others. It is important to know some basics in de-escalating a situation if this happens; these are illustrated in Figures 11.1 and 11.2.

Voice	Body language
Gentle and calm tone of voice	Open posture
Familiar words	Calm demeanour
Use their name regularly	Calm demeanour
Break down tasks into smaller steps	Smile!
One question at a time	Appropriate eye contact
Ensure understanding	Appropriate eye contact
Be positive	Go slowly and give plenty of space

Figure 11.1: Communication: voice and body language

Validation	Activity	Moving along...	Environment
'That sounds very worrying for you'	'Can you come and help me with this first?'	Example: If a patient starts asking to go home, start talking to them about home	Moving rooms
	Folding sheets		Go for a walk
'I can see you are very upset about this'	Making the bed		Pull curtains around the bed
	Filing	Where do you live?	
'I'm so sorry that you are feeling this way'	Moving (empty boxes)	What shops are nearby?	Remove obstructions
	Word quizzes		Increase/decrease light as required
	Cup of tea	Did you work nearby?	
'Is there anything you would like me to do to help?'	Food	What do you do for fun around there?	Give plenty of space
	Colouring		

Figure 11.2: Distraction

How to make best practice happen

Have I asked why Kenny is reacting this way?	Routine is important. Since he came into hospital, Kenny's routine has been broken and he is being stopped from doing what he normally does. His job is his identity and so blocking him is removing his personhood and role within his world. Kenny becomes aggressive when staff try to impose their work routine on him.
What are Kenny's strengths/ abilities?	Kenny is an active person. He is not one to sit still and read a magazine or watch television. One of Kenny's strengths is walking; he spends most of his day at home on his feet. Kenny shows his emotions through his behaviour – when he is unhappy or feeling threatened, then a strength he has is to demonstrate his upset through his behaviour. Kenny is able to hold a conversation and make jokes. He has spent his life socialising with members of the public. He is able to mobilise freely and likes to keep moving.

	Qualified staff	Healthcare support worker
Am I listening?	Kenny's behaviour is telling us that something is not right. When he is blocked, Kenny becomes aggressive but before that he is fine. Kenny wants to walk, he wants to stand near the doors and speak to people in his own way. Use a behaviour chart to monitor Kenny's reactions and learn about what triggers agitation.	Most people do not punch staff for no reason. Appreciate that something is causing Kenny to become distressed. Blocking Kenny from doing what he wants is the trigger. Familiarise yourself with Kenny's history – it will tell you why he is acting the way he is.
Do I know enough about Kenny?	Kenny was a doorman until he retired. His job is important to him. It gives a sense of purpose and identity. It was not only a job to him, but gave him a routine and developed his social life.	Asking what job Kenny did would tell you enough to understand his behaviour. If a 'This is Me' document has been filled out, familiarise yourself with it. It will tell you all you need to know about Kenny.

	Qualified staff	Healthcare support worker
What can I do to enable Kenny?	Kenny needs space to walk and benefits from standing at the main doors of the ward. Walking and standing also help Kenny with other abilities (verbal communication improves when he is in his usual routine).	Do not impose the ward routine on the patient.
		Give Kenny space to walk when he feels the need.
		Let him live out his routine as a doorman while on the ward.
	Kenny is more likely to interact with staff at the main doors, or when they are walking around the ward with him. Using his helpful nature, it may be possible to ask him to help you with certain odd jobs (such as moving boxes).	Use his mobility to promote his independence with washing, dressing and using the bathroom, but when Kenny wants to.
		Hold brief conversations with Kenny and have a joke with him. Stand with him at the door when you have a few minutes. This will help him feel comfortable on the ward and keep his mind stimulated, minimising aggressive behaviour.

Chapter 12

Frank – Environment

Frank is a 79-year-old retired builder who sustained a fall at home and has been admitted onto the surgical ward for conservative management of a pubic ramus fracture. The multidisciplinary team has managed to get his pain under control and the physiotherapist has discharged Frank as he has been mobilising independently unaided on the ward.

It has been noted that Frank is 'wandering' on the ward throughout the day and it is documented that he is difficult to settle at night time. He struggles to settle to eat his lunch, his oral intake is fluctuant and Frank has been found urinating in the hallway at times.

Frank was diagnosed with dementia ten months ago after his wife noticed he was struggling to concentrate to watch the television and he was becoming increasingly forgetful.

INTRODUCTION

Admission to an acute hospital can be distressing and disorientating for a person with dementia (Cunningham 2006) and behaviours and symptoms associated with their condition may be exacerbated as a result of the change in environment. The acute environment is designed to manage acute conditions and therefore ward design is focused on surveillance, security and infection control (Digby and Bloomer 2013). The result is many competing stimuli, which can be very stressful for the person with dementia (McCloskey 2004) and can result in agitation, withdrawal, navigation difficulties and wandering (Digby and Bloomer 2013).

People with dementia are particularly sensitive to their built and psychosocial environment (Judd, Marshall and Phippen 1998) and need a stable, consistent, familiar setting that is easy for them to negotiate and ideally reinforces their identity. Accordingly, it is not surprising that an admission to hospital can cause them enormous distress, can aggravate disorientation and precipitate challenging behaviours. The hospital environment provides multiple and competing stimuli, including noises (call bells, swinging doors, televisions, radios, trolleys), ward rounds, visitors coming and going, staff changeovers, cluttered ward layouts and poor signage, which are far from ideal for an individual with dementia. Cognitively impaired people who were functioning well in their home environment prior to hospitalisation often become extremely confused and unsettled in a general hospital setting (Thompson *et al.* 2010). Therefore, people with dementia who were living independently in their own homes prior to admission to hospital are less likely to return to their home environment following hospital discharge (MacNeill and Lichtenberg 1997). The sounds, sights, noises and smells of an acute ward can be overwhelming and frightening. In order to make this more manageable, the essence of caring for an individual with dementia is to be aware of the impact of change and the need for effective communication.

Of all the senses, hearing is the one that has the most significant impact on people with dementia in terms of their quality of life. This is due to the decline in an individual's cognitive functioning with regard to the effects of sensory changes, altering how an individual perceives noise and light. As hearing is linked to balance via the vestibular system, this can also lead to an increased risk of falls through loss of balance or an increase in disorientation as a result of people trying to orientate themselves in an over-stimulating and noisy ward.

People with dementia often respond on a sensory level rather than intellectually; for example, they will note the tone of voice or the body language of staff rather than what they say (Van Hoof *et al.* 2010). This sensitivity can change over the course of a day and can be due to a reduced ability to interpret one's sensory environment. When this is combined with age-related decline in hearing, the result is people reacting to their environment rather than being supported by it.

If other senses are overloaded at the same time as hearing (touch, sight, smell, taste), the effect can be a dramatic change in an individual's behaviour. Thus, staff often categorise mealtimes as being particularly challenging. Evidence highlights the importance of appropriate music for maximum enjoyment at mealtimes, even for people who do not have a cognitive impairment (Woods *et al.* 2011). Figure 12.1 shows how the environment can impact on a person with dementia.

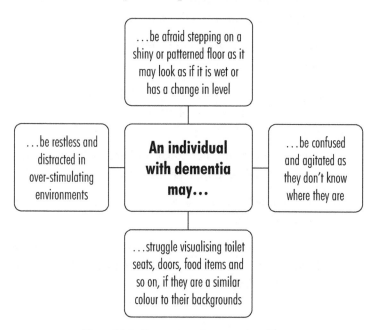

Figure 12.1: Common environmental problems

ENVIRONMENTAL GUIDELINES THAT SHOULD BE INCORPORATED INTO THE DESIGN OF A WARD

Dementia design principles should maintain independence, enhance self-esteem and confidence, demonstrate care for staff, be orientating and understandable for the patient, reinforce personal identity, welcome carers, compensate for disability and allow control of stimuli. These principles can be encompassed with the following design features:

- Clear signage outside each bed bay must be reassuring and help patients and visitors locate day rooms. Signage should incorporate a photograph, a symbol and written words, in appropriate colours to support those with visual and cognitive impairments.

- There should be coloured privacy doors to help patients orientate themselves to the ward environment.

- The flooring should contrast tonally with the furniture and the walls.

- The floor covering should not be patterned or have a pronounced speckle or sparkle to it. Make sure wood-effect vinyls do not have a strong grain effect.

- There should be no tonal difference between the flooring inside and outside the bathroom.

- At least one large clear analogue clock should be visible from all bed areas.

- The wall colour should be warm and light to maximise light levels. It should not be patterned and the finish should be matte.

- The bed areas should be made as distinct as possible. Try using different laminates, upholstery and footboard styles to make them more individualised.

- Light-coloured curtains to the bed area will provide privacy and will help keep the bed area as light as possible when the curtains are closed.

- Encourage patients to take a personal pillow, bed throw, photographs and other small items which can reassure patients and can also remind staff about the patient they are caring for.

- Ensure that there is excellent lighting in the room, both daylight and artificial. Consider the use of biodynamic LED lighting in longer-stay wards.

It is vital that staff make the most of the environment around them for their patients by:

- minimising background noise

- having signage at a patient's eye level (for example, for toilets)

- playing relaxing music in the background

- manipulating the environment to suit the person's needs (lights to the toilet at night, toilet door open)

- engaging the patient in activities of daily living

- making the bedside more homely by using their own personal items, such as pictures of their loved ones and a favourite pillow

- providing lots of reassurance and orientation to the patient to relieve any distress or confusion.

BIODYNAMIC LIGHTING

Adequate lighting is vitally important for people with dementia. For older people – with or without dementia – changes to the eye mean that less light is able to reach the retina, making it harder to see and carry out tasks.

In dementia, changes can occur in the occipital lobe, which is responsible for processing visual information. Deficits can cause blurring of the edges of objects, difficulty picking out objects that have a similar tone and difficulty understanding levels and distances, and these can all contribute to falls.

Insufficient natural light has a negative effect on health and well-being, and these effects are likely to increase during a hospital admission:

- disruption in sleep pattern
- wakefulness
- confusion
- decreased activity
- reduced alertness
- daytime napping
- mood fluctuation
- agitation
- anxiety
- depression.

Biodynamic lighting is an artificial light source controlled by a light management system to replicate the dynamic variations of daylight and sunlight (Lighting for Health 2013). It enables the body to maintain a normal circadian cycle and has positive effects on our health and well-being.

Research has shown many positive benefits of biodynamic lighting:

- It helps to set the biological clock in older adults, especially people with dementia to a 24-hour sleep/ wake cycle. Restoring the biological clock can enable people to be active throughout the day.

- It helps to increase alertness and productivity. After a restful night's sleep they have more energy to engage with activities such as gardening, playing cards, meeting and enjoying time with relatives and friends, or simply relaxing, reading, listening to music or watching TV.

- It can help to provide a more restful sleep at night and can result in a reduced requirement for night sedation.

People with dementia who are not exposed to sufficient amounts of natural daylight can benefit from a biodynamic lighting scheme as it will help them to maintain a normal sleeping pattern.

THE IMPACT OF THE SOCIAL ENVIRONMENT ON A PERSON WITH DEMENTIA

The way a person with dementia feels and experiences life is down to more than just having the condition. There are many factors aside from the symptoms of dementia that play a huge part in shaping someone's experiences. These include an individual's relationships, their environment and the support they receive.

Personal relationships and someone's social environment are central to their lives. People can recognise this by being as supportive as possible. Carers, friends and family can help a person with dementia maintain their identity and feel valued. Support should be sensitive to the person as an individual and focus on meeting their needs and promoting their well-being.

It is vital that carers have an understanding of the impact that dementia has on that person. This includes understanding how the person might think and feel, as these things will affect how they behave. The person may be experiencing a world that is very different to that of the people around them. A carer needs to offer support while seeing things from the perspective of the person with dementia. Each person is a unique individual with their own personality, preferences, dislikes and life history. It is very important to focus on what the person is able to do and not on what they are unable to do. Dementia has many effects and most individuals experience difficulties with memory and making decisions.

These in turn may lead to the loss of:

- confidence

- independence

- self-esteem

- social roles and relationships

- the ability to complete everyday activities or hobbies.

Despite losing the ability to complete these tasks, the individual will still retain some of their abilities, and will still feel an emotional connection to people and their environment, even in the advanced stages of the disease. Changes to the hospital environment do not need to be expensive or complicated. Simple improvements could include a social area, signage or easy-to-read information. These changes will lead to increased dignity and privacy for patients.

How to make best practice happen

Have I asked why Frank is reacting this way?	Is Frank agitated by the beeping infusion pump beside his bedside?
	What is Frank's daily routine? Does he normally sleep in his armchair, fall asleep to a particular TV programme, get up at 5am?
	Look and listen to what is going on in the ward near Frank. Is there anything which might be affecting him negatively?
	Can you make the environment easier for Frank to understand, with signs and positioning near the toilets?
What are Frank's strengths/ abilities?	Frank is independently mobile and likes walking outdoors. Ensure that you try to support Frank with getting outside during the day for a breath of fresh air.

	Qualified staff	Healthcare support worker
Am I listening?	Listen to what Frank is trying to tell you. Is he frightened of staff as they are strangers to him?	Has Frank altered the tone in his voice?
	Does he know where the toilet is and has he mistaken an area in the hallway as a urinal? Is he able to read the orientation board on his table?	Is he making eye contact with you or is he focusing on a particular object in his environment?
Do I know enough about Frank?	Have we asked about Frank's ambitious career. Speaking with his family would enable you to find out that Frank was the owner of a very successful construction company in the UK which his son now runs.	Familiarise yourself with Frank's social history. Encourage family/friends to engage in Frank's previous pastimes and activities. Ask Frank about his work, home life and family life.
	Who are the most important people in Frank's life?	

	Qualified staff	Healthcare support worker
What can I do to enable Frank?	Set up a lunch group in the ward with other patients. When Frank sees fellow patients sitting around the table eating, he may familiarise himself with the task of social eating that he has participated in for the majority of his life.	What is Frank's daily routine? Does he like to rise early or prefer to sleep later? Does he enjoy listening to the radio or watching TV? It may be that he prefers spending time outside, and therefore spending all day inside can be distressing and depressing, especially on warmer days.

Chapter 13

Miriam – Boredom in Hospital

Miriam is 81 years old and has a diagnosis of Alzheimer's disease. She has been admitted to hospital after fracturing her tibia in a fall. Miriam has had episodes of diarrhoea and has been placed in a side room.

Over the past few days she has been very unstable on her feet, resulting in her spending most of the time in bed. Miriam has been frequently crying out when left on her own and has fallen out of the bed twice. She is withdrawn and quiet when staff are present. She is refusing to eat her meals and she turns away when staff make attempts to care for her. Her family have visited a couple of times and confirm that these behaviours are not normal for her.

INTRODUCTION

Being in hospital is not often mentally stimulating for the patient. Plain, clinical wards, everything looking exactly the same and spending long periods of time in bed with often very repetitive conversations and actions with staff do not foster an engaging and inspiring environment. Patients often bring in activities from home to keep themselves entertained or distracted such as books, tablets or phones, but people with dementia and their carers rarely bring items to occupy them.

Dementia can decrease a person's motivation and the ability to 'entertain' themselves, leading to sensory deprivation.

Because of this, boredom can make a person with dementia appear very withdrawn and more confused. This can lead to agitation, a decline in activities of daily living and a decline in social functioning. It is highly likely that this will happen in hospital when the person with dementia is physically unwell and so more cognitively impaired as a consequence. Often wards have no social space, which results in patients being kept by their bedside or in bed for long periods of time and in many cases not knowing the reason they are there, increasing the likelihood of boredom, aggression and withdrawal.

BENEFITS OF ACTIVITY FOR THE PARTICIPANT

We all engage in activity, and we can all experience enjoyment and pleasure from this, with physical exercise having a significant impact on a person's well-being. Some other benefits include:

- maintaining skills and independence
- having the ability to express emotions
- increasing social interaction (depending on the activity)
- feeling a sense of belonging
- feeling important and valued.

The Hello Brain project research (Institute of Neuroscience, Trinity College Dublin 2014) showed that mental stimulation is the secret ingredient to staying young in mind. This involves challenging your brain, getting it to jump those mental hurdles it might shy away from. Research has shown mental activity is likely to add to brain reserve, topping up your account so that you can keep going even when faced with the threat of neurodegenerative disease (Institute of Neuroscience, Trinity College Dublin 2015).

BENEFITS TO STAFF

Activity will not just benefit the person with dementia, but can also benefit staff, whether they are participating in the activity with the person, supervising or carrying on with their work around the ward. It can:

- help to maintain a positive relationship

- provide a break from the everyday caring routine

- promote feelings of comfort and security (patient to carer)

- potentially improve challenging behaviours.

(Alzheimer's Society 2014)

THE IMPORTANCE OF KNOWING YOUR PATIENT

As was mentioned with Kenny (Chapter 11), providing activity for a patient can only be done through knowing the patient's likes, dislikes, usual routines and abilities.

Think about the time of day for the patient; if they are drowsier in the morning, then it is probably not the best time to do an activity that requires a lot of concentration, but maybe the person might like to engage in something like a hand massage or listen to some music.

With Miriam, boredom played a big part in her change of behaviour. She felt isolated and cut off in the side room. There was no stimulation and no effort to provide anything from the clinical staff. Her family were also unsure about what Miriam was allowed or able to do and so the situation just worsened.

When a healthcare support worker gave the family a 'This is Me' form to complete, it opened up a wide range of activities and topics of conversation for staff and Miriam. Miriam used to be an artist; she painted watercolour scenes, made clay sculptures and was also a singer in some local clubs. Using this information, ward staff were able to suggest that her family brought in her watercolours for her to paint (unfortunately, Miriam was unable to use them as she used to since the activity was too challenging for her degree of cognitive impairment). Instead, the ward used Aquapaint (Active Minds 2016), a picture that can be 'painted' with water and disappears when dry. Miriam was also give some play dough, which she would squash in her hands and roll into balls as if she was using clay.

TIPS ON STARTING AN ACTIVITY

These tips will help with starting an activity. They do not need to be followed for each person with dementia, but can help guide the activities that are chosen.

- Activities should be stimulating but should not involve too many challenges or choices.

- Concentration may be reduced, so consider short bursts of activity.

- If the person is not interested, come back later or try a different activity.

- Break down instructions and make steps simple.

- Consider easy, repetitive actions.

- 'Normal', everyday life activities can help people feel useful and valued.

- Focus on enjoyment and participation rather than achievement.

- Consider the optimum time of day for the individual.

- Use demonstration and support the individual through difficult parts.

- Help with task initiation.

- Encourage creativity and self-expression.

- Let the person know how well they are doing and how much they are needed.

For Miriam, just having the activity placed in front of her was enough. She was able to pick up a brush or the play dough and engage in the activity independently. As her dementia progresses, her ability to self-entertain will decrease and it may be that at times staff will need to place objects into her hand, or, as things progress further, Miriam may enjoy the act of watching someone else paint.

HAS THE ACTIVITY BEEN HELPFUL?

The most important measure of how 'helpful' an activity has been is how happy the person is. Activity can mean that relationships between patients and staff are strengthened, which can in turn lead to reduction in anxiety and agitation, and quite possibly to some physical changes – sitting out of bed more, perhaps walking more, improving sleep patterns.

There was a global improvement in Miriam's mood and ability to engage and interact with the staff after she had been involved in activity. She looked forward to new activity and was pleased to see staff coming into her room.

How to make best practice happen

Have I asked why Miriam is reacting this way?	The 'why' for Miriam was boredom and isolation. This is always going to be a challenge in hospital but it can be overcome with the support of clinical teams and families. Step into Miriam's shoes and ask yourself how you would feel, isolated in a strange place with nothing to do for 24 hours a day.	
What are Miriam's strengths/ abilities?	Miriam is able to demonstrate through her behaviour that she is not happy. She is able to join in with basic painting and playing with play dough. If we spend a little time looking at our patients, even those with very advanced dementia still show emotion – it is so important that we notice this strength and respond to it accordingly. Miriam shows enjoyment when she is doing something she likes. Miriam likes to be tactile and hold hands.	

	Qualified staff	**Healthcare support worker**
Am I listening?	Miriam is withdrawn, disengaged and agitated from time to time. Her family have told us her behaviour is not normal. What is her normal behaviour? How does she act when she is upset?	What is making Miriam sad on occasion? Try different approaches to cheering her up. Her withdrawn behaviour is a communication – what is she trying to tell you?
Do I know enough about Miriam?	Does your patient have a 'This is Me' form? What do they like to do for enjoyment? What upsets them?	Look at the 'This is Me' form; what are Miriam's likes and dislikes? What activities or resources are available on the ward that can be used to engage Miriam?

| What can I do to enable Miriam? | Showing emotion, either positive or negative is a strength that patients with dementia have and that we can use. Spend some time trying different activities with Miriam to see which one elicits a positive emotion.

Use Miriam's expertise and artistic talent to choose suitable activities. | Ensure that Miriam's favourite pastimes of painting and playing with play dough are built into her daily routine on the ward.

Set up the task on her bedside table, ensure that she can reach all the objects and is able to initiate the task independently. Engage Miriam in familiar activities such as music or television, which will occupy her when she is on her own in the side room.

Miriam may also respond well to a gentle exercise such as a hand massage, which can be done in bed or in a chair. |

Chapter 14

Nicky and Denise – Approaching the End of Life

Nicky is 52 years old and was diagnosed with vascular dementia eight years ago. Nicky's wife Denise has been her main carer for the past four years, and they have a daughter called Kit. Nicky was very independent after her diagnosis and was able to continue working as a teacher for five years. She took early retirement as she began to have significant word-finding difficulties and her concentration was affected as a result of sustaining a number of transient ischemic attacks (TIAs). A care package was commenced at this time and has gradually increased to having two carers visit four times a day to support with personal care and meals. She attends a specialist day centre for people with young onset dementia twice a week, but they have started to struggle to manage her physical needs, in particular mobility and eating.

This morning the carers could not get Nicky out of bed. Denise had noticed that Nicky's breathing had changed, she looked clammy and she was trying to cough. Denise called the ambulance and Nicky has been taken to hospital.

HOW A PERSON WITH DEMENTIA MIGHT DIE

Dementia shortens life expectancy, but it is a challenge to know how long a person will live for once diagnosed. There are many factors that can have an impact on the speed of the progression:

- the physical and mental health of the person

- genetics

- other comorbidities a person might have, which may deteriorate in a more predictable way and shorten a person's life before the dementia has an impact

- age at diagnosis – generally, if dementia is diagnosed before the age of 65 there is a more rapid deterioration

- the support networks that are in place around an individual.

Nicky was diagnosed with dementia when she was 44 years old, and other than her dementia she was a very healthy person, she enjoyed the outdoors with her family and had a good level of fitness. She wanted to live well with her dementia and remained positive and proactive in her approach to life, with the support of her wife and daughter. Nicky deteriorated relatively slowly, but there were changes; she suffered frequent migraines which indicated that she was having TIAs. The most significant changes occurred in the past year when she became doubly incontinent, her mobility deteriorated significantly, she struggled to communicate verbally and often became frustrated and tearful. More recently, it was evident that she was developing problems with swallowing.

It is important to know when a person with dementia is reaching the end of their life so that the right treatment and services can be provided and the family have an opportunity to work through the emotional impact of the situation. When Nicky was admitted to hospital, Denise wanted to know whether her wife was coming towards the end of her life, but this can be a difficult question to answer. Eychmuller, Constantini and Domeisen (2012) explain that actually diagnosing dying is challenging because there is no common definition of the dying phase in dementia. It can be particularly difficult to determine for people with dementia as a person may be at the end-stage of dementia for some time, but not in the dying phase. The length of time the person experiences end-stage dementia can vary hugely, from months to a few years. The symptoms listed below are adapted from the *End-of-life care* factsheet from the Alzheimer's Society (2014) and indicate when a person is reaching the end stage of dementia:

- memory loss, failing to recognise loved ones, perhaps their own reflection

- reduced eating and drinking; associated swallowing problems and weight loss

- limited speech, perhaps one-word answers or no speech at all, but non-verbal communication may still be used to show needs and feelings

- incontinence, bowel and urinary

- little or no independent function, unable to walk or stand, problems sitting up and becoming bed-bound

- needing support with most, possibly all, activities of daily living.

Dementia is a life-limiting illness, and death usually occurs as a result of complications arising from the effects of the disease rather than the disease itself. The complication is likely to be listed on the death certificate as cause of death, with dementia being an associated cause.

APPROACHING DEMENTIA AS A TERMINAL ILLNESS

Shortly after she was diagnosed, Nicky made a Lasting Power of Attorney for her personal welfare, with Denise as the attorney.

Nicky wanted to discuss her wishes openly and honestly while she was still able to make informed decisions so that Denise could then support them if she lost capacity. She also did not want her to feel guilty. Decisions about future care needs should be discussed as part of an ongoing process from the time of diagnosis onwards, so people with dementia can feel confident that their preferences and wishes can be acted on. Advanced care plans or advanced decisions to refuse a specific medical treatment can support the person with dementia and family carers, and give clarity when there are difficult and challenging decisions to be made.

Early discussions about possible future scenarios may feel wrong, but it is essential that we give people with dementia the opportunity to express their wishes as their future self may not be able to do this, particularly when their care needs become palliative. However, the Social Care Institute for Excellence (2015) highlights that most people with dementia have not made these formal arrangements, and family carers are then drawn into making decisions at times when they are probably at their most distressed.

In recent years the National End of Life Care Strategy (Department of Health 2008), the National Dementia Strategy (Department of Health 2009) and the Prime Minister's Challenge (Department of Health 2012) have all highlighted the importance of planning end-of-life care for people with dementia and there is a call for continued and significant improvements to be made. There is now a recognition that people with dementia should have full access to palliative care services and this is particularly important as the ethos of palliative care complements the aims of person-centred dementia care.

Understanding the differences between advance care plans, advance decisions, statement of wishes and preferences and Lasting Powers of Attorney can be challenging and easy to mix up, but Figure 14.1, taken from the National End of Life Team, summarises the definitions.

Advance care planning

ACP is a process of discussion between an individual and their care providers irrespective of discipline.

The difference between ACP and planning more generally is that the process of ACP is to make clear a person's wishes and will usually take place in the context of an anticipated deterioration in the individual's condition in the future, with attendant loss of capacity to make decision and/or ability to communicate wishes to others.

With the individual's agreement, discussions should be:

- documented
- regularly reviewed
- communicated to key persons involved in their care.

Examples of what an ACP discussion might include are:

- the individual's concerns
- their important values of personal goals for care
- their understanding about their illness and prognosis, as well as particular preferences for types of care or treatment that may be beneficial in the future and the availability of these.

Statement of Wishes and Preferences

This is a summary term embracing a range of written and/or recorded oral expressions, by which people can, if they wish, write down or tell people about their wishes or preferences in relation to future treatment or care, or explain their feelings, beliefs and values that govern how they make decisions. They may cover medical and non-medical matters. They are not legally binding but should be used when determining a person's best interests in the event they lose capacity to make those decisions.

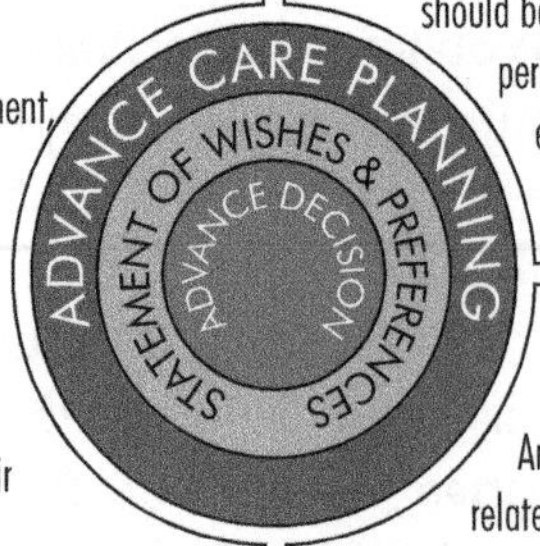

Advance decision

An advance decision must relate to a refusal of specific medical treatment and can specify circumstances.

It will come into effect when the individual has lost capacity to give or refuse consent to treatment.

Careful assessment of the validity and applicability of an advance decision is essential before it is used in clinical practice. Valid advance decisions, which are refusals of treatment, are legally binding.

Lasting Power of Attorney

A Lasting Power of Attorney (LPA) is a statutory form of power of attorney created by the MCA (2005). Anyone who has the capacity to do so may choose a person (an attorney) to take decisions on their behalf if they subsequently lose capacity.

Figure 14.1: Advance Care Planning: A Guide for Health and Social Care Staff (National End of Life Team 2008)

LOSS AND GRIEVING (FOR THE CARER)

Loss and grief are usually associated with the death of a loved one, but these feelings can be experienced by the carer while someone is still living, and this is sometimes called a living bereavement. This is a normal process often experienced with long-term chronic disease and it is natural for the carer to experience loss and grief throughout the journey as well as after their loved one has passed away. A carer may experience many different types of loss and the experience will be unique to their situation. Denise struggled with being called a carer; she explained, 'It was the hardest thing. Nicky is my wife and my friend and we have a beautiful daughter. When did I lose all this to be seen as just her carer?' Denise experienced this quite early on and she fought against it as she did not want her role as a wife to change.

The Family Caregiver Alliance (2013) website explains that it is easy for carers to ignore their losses and just keep doing things; they highlight that this can lead to grief, and grief can lead to sadness, depression, anger, guilt and sleeplessness and other physical and emotional problems. It is important to identify the losses that come with long-term chronic illness, so that there is an opportunity to grieve. Carers may not always have the opportunity to do this and the emotions can build up to the point where they feel depressed, angry or upset, and these emotions may play out in conversations with clinicians. It is essential that staff do not take this personally, but rather consider the context of the situation and appreciate the level of distress the carer is experiencing. Allowing carers an opportunity to talk things through is essential.

DIFFICULT CONVERSATIONS

Caring for a person with dementia is difficult at any point of the journey, but Davies et al. (2014) point out that it's potentially more difficult at the end of life because of the complex decisions that need to be made. As already discussed, an advance care plan or an advance decision to refuse treatment can give clarity when a difficult decision needs be made, but unfortunately most people with dementia have not made these arrangements. They may not have had the opportunity to discuss and formulate these plans at an early stage or they may have chosen not to enter into these discussions and will rely on their main family carer. In these situations, discussions about treatment options will be in the context of the Mental Capacity Act and a best-interests decision will be made (see Chapter 4). In all cases, however, whether or not there is an advance care plan or advance decision, conversations with the main carer around a decision whether or not to treat will be difficult and challenging, and they can be emotionally and professionally demanding. When initially breaking bad news, consider the following:

• Find a private place.

• Be sensitive, but be honest.

• Make sure you know the patient and have a plan that you can clearly lay out.

• Provide them with written information.

• Be aware that the main carer may want to meet again, so give them the opportunity to do this.

The doctors may lead on such conversations, but the main carer will potentially engage with other clinicians on the ward as they may need further clarity about the care their loved one is receiving. Chapter 2 discusses the triangle of care and recognises the importance of engaging with both the person with dementia and their main carer, but it is likely at the end-of-life stage that the conversation about treatment will remain with the carer.

Just be with them and allow them the opportunity to talk through their fears and worries. It is sometimes just helpful having someone who is really listening and understanding the emotion behind the distress. You may find some questions easy to answer, but others may be more complex and you may need the support of another clinician to provide clarity, and it is fine to say this.

DECISIONS ABOUT NUTRITION AND HYDRATION

As Nicky's disease progressed, she developed a problem with swallowing. The prevalence of swallowing problems (dysphagia) is high in people with dementia (Rösler *et al.* 2015). It is more common in advanced dementia and is often an indicator that a person is approaching the end of life.

In a person with dementia the ability to eat and drink is a complex issue and intrinsically linked to the person and the family's perception of dementia and whether they understand the life-limiting nature of the disease. The person and the family will often associate the fact that the person is unable to swallow with an episode of acute illness and believe that it can be treated and cured.

In people who have conditions complicated by factors such as stroke, swallowing difficulties might manifest themselves at an earlier stage. An acute illness can also exacerbate swallowing problems (see Table 14.1) and it is often at this point or when a person has been admitted with an aspiration pneumonia that a problem is identified.

The clinician must ensure that the reversible causes of swallowing problems have been excluded before considering that the problem might be due to the person's dementia. Early involvement of a speech and language therapist as well as a dietician should be sought.

**Table 14.1: Common causes of swallowing
difficulties in a person with dementia**

Acute	Chronic
Oral thrush/oral or dental infection	Persisting dysphagia post cerebrovascular accident
Infection, e.g. UTI	
Decline in consciousness due to acute episode of illness	Oesophageal stricture or tumour
	Parkinson's disease
Acute neurological event, e.g. cerebrovascular accident/TIA	Other progressive neurological conditions, e.g. motor neuron disease, multiple sclerosis, bulbar palsy
Medication (antipsychotics, sedatives, anticholinergics)	
Oesophageal foreign body, e.g. false teeth	Decline in consciousness as part of chronic cognitive decline or delirium
	End-of-life disease progression
	Depression (loss of appetite, food refusal or abnormal perception of food)

USE OF TUBE FEEDING

Prior to the 1980s and the introduction of fine-bore naso-gastric tubes (NG) and percutaneous endoscopic gastrostomy tubes (PEG), people with dementia would be risk fed until they died. However, there was a drive to use tube feeding when the new technology came in, particularly in nursing homes in the United States. This has led to a continued expectation of 'treatment' when a person stops swallowing effectively.

However, a Cochrane Systematic Review found no evidence that tube feeding patients with advanced dementia prolonged survival, improved quality of life, led to better nourishment or decreased the risk of pressure sores. The review suggested that it might increase the risk of pneumonia through aspiration (Sampson, Candy and Jones 2009).

Evans, Smith and Morrow (2009) identified questions that should be asked by the clinician when considering whether tube feeding would be suitable for a person with advanced dementia:

- What are you expecting to achieve?

- Are these expectations realistic?

- Has adequate information been shared with relatives and carers to ensure that they do not have unrealistic expectations of what tube feeding can achieve?

- What would the person with advanced dementia have wanted?

- Is tube feeding really in the person with advanced dementia's best interests?

- Will the benefits of human contact and stimulation from food (during all meals, snacks and drinks) be lost?

There is evidence that people at the end of life are less aware of hunger and thirst and can gain comfort from minimal intake and that most will patients die comfortably without artificial hydration (Partridge and Campbell 2007).

WHAT CAN BE DONE?

There is rarely justification for the use of tube feeding in a patient with advanced dementia; however, families and carers can struggle to come to terms with the decision not to feed a person. For Denise, the idea of letting the person she loved 'starve' felt completely unacceptable at first, in spite of the fact that Nicky had been clear about her wishes. It was important for the clinical staff to make it clear that the onus was not on Denise to make the decision and that it would be made in Nicky's best interests. Denise was allowed time to ask questions and to process the information she was being given. This helped her come to terms with the fact that Nicky was dying and the treatment that she required was supportive rather than aggressive.

Evidence shows that careful feeding (often called risk feeding) is the most appropriate approach to take and the family can be involved in this, as research has shown that it is more successful if the patient has a good relationship with the person feeding them. Denise was shown how to risk feed Nicky and they were able to spend pleasurable time together. It is thought that, nutritionally, patients fed in this way do as well as those who are tube fed.

How to make best practice happen

Have I asked why Nicky/ Denise are reacting this way?	Nicky is dying, her speech is limited, she has a significant problem with swallowing and she is sleeping for most of the time. Denise is very distressed and tearful because of the changes in her wife. The doctors have confirmed that Nicky now needs 'comfort management'.	
What are Nicky/ Denise's strengths/ abilities?	Denise has an affectionate and intimate relationship with Nicky. Denise is still able to communicate with Nicky and help to explain what she wants from staff. Nicky can still smile and sometimes laughs when music is playing. They have a loving family.	

	Qualified staff	**Healthcare support worker**
Am I listening?	Allow Denise time to talk. It is important that she has an opportunity to share her thoughts and feelings. Denise can act as Nicky's advocate as she is closest to her. Does Denise want to help with her wife's care?	Listen to what Denise tells you about Nicky. Pick up on non-verbal communication from Nicky to get a sense of how she is feeling. Is there anything you can do to make it easier for Nicky and Denise? It is often small things that matter at times like this.

Do I know enough about Nicky/ Denise?	Denise has brought Nicky's Life Story Book to the ward so that staff can get to know her and her family. The book has lots of details about their life together and the things she likes to do. Nicky loves Robbie Williams, so a CD player is organised.	Ask Nicky whether she would like to see the hospital chaplain; this would address Nicky's spiritual needs. Ensure that Nicky's music is played regularly.
What can I do to enable Nicky/ Denise?	Nicky is now much more dependent for her activities of daily living so Denise wants to support her wife and develop new skills. Show Denise some simple hand massage techniques to use on her wife. Support Denise in developing her caring skills and also be aware that she may find this very challenging and she may be upset and need to talk through the changes in her wife.	Ensure that Nicky's wife and daughter have been given a carer's passport. Nicky will not be able to tolerate too many visitors at the one time. As Nicky's ability to eat and drink reduces, she will require regular mouth care, which the healthcare support worker can show her family how to do.

Chapter 15

Stan – Touch

Stan has been admitted to the medical assessment unit (MAU) at his local hospital with breathing problems and is being treated for a chest infection. He has had dementia for several years, but it has never been formally diagnosed. His wife, Betty, explained that over the past year she has noticed a decline in husband's cognitive level; he has become slower, more forgetful and less engaged in life. Betty feels that in past week Stan has deteriorated considerably, has become more insular and uncommunicative. Since admission this has become more of a concern as Stan is only eating and drinking when Betty assists him. Despite commencing antibiotics, Stan remains disengaged and he sleeps most of the time. Betty is devastated that Stan has become so unwell in such a short space of time and she is concerned that she will not be able to support him at home.

WHY IS TOUCH IMPORTANT?

Touch is our first sense to develop and is a basic human need throughout life. The amount and type of touch we receive varies at different stages of life, but throughout it is a powerful means of communication.

> In recent years, a wave of studies has documented some incredible emotional and physical health benefits that come from touch. This research is suggesting that touch is truly fundamental to human communication, bonding, and health. (Keltner 2010)

When thinking about the human life cycle, we are touched the most as children. As part of care needs that change as we are growing and developing, and also as part of bonding with our parents, love and affection are demonstrated through holding, hugging and kissing and through play. A parent will attend to their child's care needs in a practical way, but it is likely that they will show physical love and tenderness to their child.

As we grow and develop into adults, we move on to relationships with our partners and touch is central to our loving sexual relationships; of course, the amount and level of touch can vary over time, dependent on personal circumstances and choice. When we move into older age, it is a time when we are touched the least – we may have lost our partner, our children may have grown up and live far away – but interestingly the need for touch increases. Burnside (1973) suggested that touch helps elderly people compensate for bereavement, dependency and altered body image.

There has been much criticism about the quality of many of the studies around touch that have taken place; however, the emerging research does suggest that it is beneficial and safe (Goldschmidt and van Meines 2012). The most common findings suggest that when touch is used in a therapeutic way it can:

- reduce stress and anxiety
- provide comfort and connection
- lessen pain
- improve quality of life
- offer an opportunity to unwind and relax for the giver and the receiver.

Stan was transferred to the care of the elderly ward on his third day, and although Betty was upset about the move she understood that the ward would be more suited to her husband's needs. Cranford ward was much quieter than the busy admissions ward and the environment seemed much more relaxed. Lynsey, a healthcare support worker, supported Stan into an armchair from the wheelchair. She asked him what he liked to be called while she crouched down so that he could easily see her face and she could make eye contact; smiling, she squeezed his hand, and he smiled back at her.

HOW CAN TOUCH BE USED TO SUPPORT COMMUNICATION

Lynsey's interaction with Stan demonstrates how she has used both her verbal and non-verbal skills (see Chapter 5), with touch being an integral part of this. Cognitive impairment due to dementia and the impact of a hospital admission due to illness can severely reduce the normal use of language, and this may show as an increase in stress and levels of frustration in the patient. This may lead to increased anxiety and possibly behaviours that we find challenging (see Chapter 11).

Family carers' usual verbal communication patterns with their loved ones will change over time to compensate for the loss of language in the person with dementia, and you may find it helpful to discuss this with the patient's family. Goldschmidt and Van Meines (2011, p.37) acknowledge this by explaining:

> You will begin to pay more attention to the subtle changes in people and recognise the support they need and respond in a caring and thoughtful way. You will attach more significance to the flicker of light in the eyes, the rhythm of breath, or the squeeze of one's hand to indicate awareness.

Stan was diagnosed with a hypoactive delirium, and Lynsey explained to Betty that when patients struggle to communicate verbally and seem unresponsive it can be helpful to make a connection using touch. Lynsey suggested a hand massage and asked if this is something that Stan would like. Betty explained that Stan is a loving and warm man; he generally hugged his friends, and would really appreciate her trying. She also said that Stan looked more 'with it' when staff held his hand; it seemed to help him focus on what they were saying and on the immediate task. Lynsey agreed with this and described Stan as much more engaged.

WAYS TO INCORPORATE TOUCH INTO CARE SITUATIONS

We touch our patients all the time; we support them with their personal hygiene and with mobilising, and we tend to focus on the task in hand, rather than focusing on our patient and communicating that we care through our actions. Rather than concentrating on our work as a matter of routine, we should consider the emotional impact we have on our patients. This can be maximised by:

- engaging on an emotional level with those we are caring for, so we create a therapeutic relationship between ourselves and our patients

- giving ourselves time to be in the moment with our patient and get a genuine sense of what is happening. This also allows us to have a more person-centred approach as we have time to recognise the nuances of what our patients are telling us.

Stan was agitated, restless and resistive to personal care when on the admission ward, but in the days following his move to Cranford ward he became more settled. The reasons for this are multifactorial; however, it was evident that Stan responded well to the staff when his hand was held. He also appreciated being greeted with a cuddle; he developed a very strong relationship with Lynsey and called her 'my favourite girl'. Of course, Stan's care was shared by the ward staff, but he felt a close bond with Lynsey as she has been allocated to him for the first three days of his stay on Cranford ward.

SIMPLE HAND MASSAGE

Hand massage can last as long as the time you have, from a couple of minutes to half an hour. The hand massage described here is just an example; it provides a framework, but not all sessions will encompass every movement, and you may find that simply holding a patient's hand is enough for them. When Lynsey first met Stan, she held his hand and spoke to him gently and this was how things started. When she found out from Betty that Stan was 'touchy feely', she then engaged him with a simple hand massage. Betty took to massaging Stan's feet before she left each evening and this enabled Stan to relax and sleep well on the ward.

CONTRAINDICATIONS

On rare occasions, there might be contraindications to giving a patient a massage such as:

- arthritis

- osteoporosis

- open wounds, cuts and bruising

- tumours

- eczema

- broken bones

- inflammation

- sepsis.

It might be that you need to give more careful thought about what you do; for example, with arthritis you would avoid direct pressure over the joints.

CONSENT

First, ask the patient if they would like a hand massage. If the patient is unable to respond due to communication difficulties or not understanding what you are asking, then try holding their hand and see how they respond. Continue to explain what you intend to do, speaking softly and calmly. It might also be helpful to play some relaxing music, creating a calming atmosphere. Then, if the person does not move their hand away, gently stroke it using your thumb. Again you may want to discuss hand massage with the patient's family, as some people are naturally 'touchy feely' and others will be averse to touch. It is also worth noting that preferences for touch may change with the progression of dementia; people previously averse may begin to communicate in a more non-verbal way, and touch may become an integral part of this.

Your skills will develop as you perform and it's something you can practise on friends and family. A hand massage can be as simple as holding hands and gently stroking, or a more complex routine as described below.

THINGS YOU MAY NEED

- Small pillow or cushion (you may be able to use the patient's).

- A chair so that you are comfortable – the patient may want to stay in bed or use a comfortable chair.

- A small towel or some paper towels to protect the pillow and clothes.

- Soft background music, if possible, to reduce the impact of the noise on the ward.

THINGS TO DO

- Remove jewellery and store it safely.

- Wash your hands and those of the patient.

- Roll their sleeves up to the elbow.

- Warm your hands by rubbing them together (or warm them under the hot tap when washing them).

- Sit so that you are facing each other and use pillows to make sure the arms and hand are supported.

- Ensure that you are both comfortable.

BACK OF HAND

Warm either massage oil or a hand cream in your hands and then gently apply enough on the hands and arms upwards in long and gentle strokes, ensuring that your hand moulds to the shape of the person receiving the massage. Figure 15.1 shows how holding the patient's hand can help as it supports the hand and the arm.

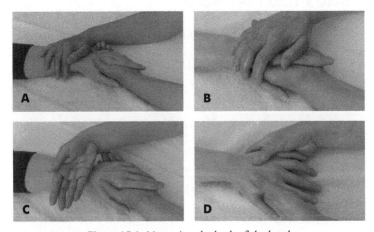

Figure 15.1: Massaging the back of the hand

Use large half-circular strokes from the centre to the side of the hand; again support the patient's hand with your hands. Then with your thumbs, using a light pressure, make little 'o' shapes over the back of the hand and around the wrist area.

PALM OF HAND

Figure 15.2 demonstrates how to support the hand while working on the palm. Your fingers slot in with the patients fingers and then you use your thumbs to complete the strokes. If you feel that this would not work with your patient, hold the patient's hand with your hand and then massage with the other, using short-/medium-length strokes from wrist to fingertips with moderate pressure. Gently lift the tissue of the entire palm using moderate pressure. Again use small circular strokes over the entire palm with moderate pressure, making little 'o' shapes. Then use large half-circular stretching strokes from centre of the palm to the sides using moderate pressure.

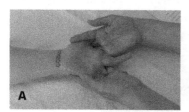
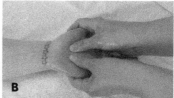

Figure 15.2: Massaging the palm of the hand

WRIST

Supporting the hand with your fingers, use your thumbs to gently work around the wrist area with gentle strokes and little 'o' shapes. You can work your way up the arm with one hand, using the other hand to continue to support the patient's hand and arm.

FINGER MASSAGE

Gently squeeze the fingers from the base to the tip on both sides and top/bottom using light pressure (as shown in Figure 15.3). Then use a gentle circular range of motion of each finger followed by a gentle squeeze of the nail bed.

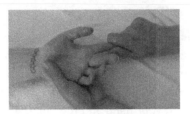

Figure 15.3: Massaging the fingers

COMPLETION OF THE HAND MASSAGE

Lay the person's hand on yours and cover it with your hand. Gently draw your top hand towards you several times (Figure 15.4). Turn the person's hand over and gently draw the other hand towards you several times. If you have a towel available, wrap the hand in the towel before you move on the other hand.

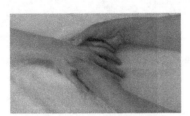

Figure 15.4: Finishing the massage

How to make best practice happen

Have I asked why Stan is reacting this way?	Stan has a hypoactive delirium due to his chest infection. Stan is confused and disorientated and needs to have lots of reality orientation; ask him why he is not eating and find out what his likes and dislikes are.	
What are Stan's strengths/ abilities?	Stan is tactile and responds well to touch. Stan is able to show affection. Stan is a very friendly character and loves to be around people.	
	Qualified staff	**Healthcare support worker**
Am I listening?	Betty explained that Stan deteriorated considerably in the week prior to his admission – he was no longer talking and he was disengaged from what was going on around him.	When the healthcare support worker spoke with Betty, she found out about how Stan normally functions in his everyday life. Betty reported that Stan was able to mobilise short distances indoors with his walking stick and is usually a humorous and chatty gentleman. The healthcare support worker was able to inform the doctor that this 'insular, uncommunicative' presentation was not normal for Stan.
Do I know enough about Stan?	When he was moved to Cranford ward, staff spent time with both Stan and Betty so they could find out his likes and dislikes. Lynsey found out that Stan was 'touchy feely' and held his hand when talking with him.	Ask Betty to complete the 'This is Me' form to outline what Stan likes and dislikes, his sensory impairments, and so on.

	Qualified staff	Healthcare support worker
What can I do to enable Stan?	When staff communicate with Stan, holding his hand has helped him focus.	Ensure that you hold Stan's hand when you are talking to him.
	Stan has responded well to staff hugging him when they have finished their shifts, and this then led to Stan talking and engaging socially.	When Stan is anxious, try physical contact, such as a hand massage.
	Staff found out that Stan liked country music, in particular Dolly Parton, so they found a CD for him to listen to and he would dance.	Maximise his social skills by including Stan in as much conversation as possible.
		Encourage Betty to give Stan a hand massage when she visits as this will enable her to interact with her husband.
	Betty expressed that being able to massage Stan's hands allowed them to keep a sense of intimacy, and she feels that this helped his recovery.	Ensure that there is a radio available to Stan to play his favourite music.

List of Tables and Figures

Bibliography

Abbey, J., Piller, N., De Bellis, A., Esterman, A. *et al.* (2004) 'The Abbey Pain Scale: a 1-minute numerical indicator for people with end-stage dementia.' *International Journal of Palliative Nursing 10*, 1, 6–13.

Active minds (2016) *Aquapaint.* London: Active minds. Accessed on 13/06/2016 at www.active-minds.co.uk/shop/dementia-art-activities/aquapaint

Age UK (2016) Factsheet 76: *Intermediate Care and Reablement.* London: Age UK. Accessed on 20/08/2016 at www.ageuk.org.uk/Documents/EN-GB/Factsheets/FS76_Intermediate_care_and_re-ablement_fcs.pdf?dtrk=true

Allan, K., McLean, F. and Scott Gibson, L. (2016) *Dementia and Deafness.* Edinburgh: Deaf Action.

Alzheimer's Europe (2009) *Position Paper on the Use of Advance Directives.* [online] Luxembourg: eZ Publish. Accessed on 17/06/2016 at www.alzheimer-europe.org/Policy-in-Practice2/Our-opinion-on/Advance-directives

Alzheimer's Society (2009) *Counting the Cost.* London: Alzheimer's Society. Accessed on 29/04/2016 at www.alzheimers.org.uk/countingthecost

Alzheimer's Society (2012) *Deprivation of Liberty Safeguards (DoLS).* London: Alzheimer's Society. Accessed on 20/05/2016 at www.alzheimers.org.uk/site/scripts/documents_info.php?documentID=1327

Alzheimer's Society (2013) *Anti-psychotic Drugs.* London: Alzheimer's Society. Accessed on 19/06/2016 at www.alzheimers.org.uk/site/scripts/documents_info.php?documentID=548

Alzheimer's Society (2014) *Staying Involved and Active.* London: Alzheimer's Society. Accessed on 22/06/2016 at www.alzheimers.org.uk/site/scripts/documents_info.php?documentID=115

Alzheimer's Society (2014) *Advice for Nurses and Other Healthcare Professionals.* London: Alzheimer's Society. Accessed on 11/07/2016 at www.alzheimers.org.uk/site/scripts/documents_info.php?documentID=1211&pageNumber=2

Alzheimer's Society (2014) *End-of-life Care.* London: Alzheimer's Society. Accessed on 07/07/2016 at www.alzheimers.org.uk/site/scripts/documents_info.php?documentID=2709

Alzheimer's Society (2014) *Lasting Power of Attorney*. London: Alzheimer's Society. Accessed on 14/06/2016 at www.alzheimers.org.uk/site/scripts/documents_info.php?documentID=154

Alzheimer's Society (2014) *Statistical Infographic*. London: Alzheimer's Society. Accessed on 16/07/2016 at https://s3.amazonaws.com/14078_Alzheimers_Interactive_Infographic/pdf/as_downloadable_infographics.pdf

Alzheimer's Society (2016) *Communicating*. London: Alzheimer's Society. Accessed on 27/05/2016 at www.alzheimers.org.uk/site/scripts/documents_info.php?documentID=130

American Geriatrics Society, Panel on Persistent Pain in Older Persons (2002) 'The management of persistent pain in older persons.' *Journal of American Geriatric Society 50*, 6, 205–224.

Archibald, C. (2006) 'Meeting the nutritional needs of patients with dementia in hospital.' *Nursing Standard 20*, 45, 41–45.

Barulich, A., Rizzardi, K. and Sunden, K. (2012) *Paper 28 'Sleep Hygiene in Hospitalized Adults' Pharmacy and Nursing Student Research and Evidence-Based Medicine Poster Session*. Cedarville, OH: Cedarville University. Accessed on 18/05/2016 at http://digitalcommons.cedarville.edu/cgi/viewcontent.cgi?article=1044&context=pharmacy_nursing_poster_session

Beauchamp, T. and Childress, J. (2009) *Principles of Biomedical Ethics, 6th Edition*. New York and Oxford: Oxford University Press.

Blackhall, A., Hawkes, D., Hingley, D. and Wood, S. (2011) 'VERA framework: communicating with people who have dementia.' *Nursing Standard 26*, 10, 35–39.

Brenner, T. and Brenner, K. (2012) *You Say Goodbye and We Say Hello: The Montessori Method for Positive Dementia Care*. Chicago, IL: Brenner Pathways.

British Dental Association (2013) *Dental Problems and Their Management in Patients with Dementia. BDA Evidence Summary*. London: BDA.

British Geriatrics Society (2014) *Fit for Frailty – Consensus for Best Practice Guidance for the Care of Older People Living in Community and Outpatients Settings*. London: British Geriatric Society. Accessed on 06/07/2016 at www.bgs.org.uk/campaigns/fff/fff_full.pdf

British Geriatrics Society (2015) *Fit for Frailty – Part 2 – Developing, Commissioning and Managing Services for People Living with Frailty in Community Settings*. London: British Geriatric Society. Accessed on 09/04/2016 at www.bgs.org.uk/campaigns/fff/fff2_full.pdf

Burnside, I. (1973) 'Touching is talking.' *American Journal of Nursing 73*, 12, 2060–2063.

Cambridge University Hospitals NHS Foundation Trust (2014) *Brief Encounters*. Cambridge: Cambridge University Hospitals NHS Foundation Trust. Accessed on 11/04/2016 at www.brief-encounters.org/?doing_wp_cron=1472558608.7727448940277099609375

Care Services Efficiency Delivery Programme: Homecare Re-ablement Workstream (2007) *Homecare Re-ablement Retrospective Longitudinal Study.* London: Care Services Efficiency Delivery. Accessed on 13/08/2016 at www.lincolnshire.gov.uk/upload/public/attachments/938/longitudinal_study__homecare_reablement.pdf

Charalambous, L. (2016) 'Implementing change in older people's acute care.' *Nursing Times 112,* 27/28, 15–17.

Clarke, A. and Bright, L. (2002) *Showing Restraint: Challenging the Use of Restraint in Care Homes.* London: Counsel & Care.

Cohen-Mansfield, J. (2000) 'Nonpharmacological management of behavioural problems in persons with dementia: the TREAT model.' *Alzheimer Care Quarterly 1, 4,* 22–34.

Cunningham, C. (2006) 'Understanding challenging behaviour in patients with dementia.' *Nursing Standard 20,* 47, 42–45.

Davies, N., Maio, I., Rait, G. and Iliffe, S. (2014) 'Quality end-of-life care for dementia: What have family carers told us so far? A narrative synthesis.' *Palliative Medicine 28,* 7, 919–930.

Dementia Action Alliance (2012) *Dementia Care in Acute Hospitals: A Report from the Dementia Action Alliance South Central Region.* London: NHS Institute for Innovation and Improvement. Accessed on 19/03/2016 at www.dementiaaction.org.uk/assets/0000/1757/CHKS_South_Central_Region_Report.pdf

Dementia Services Development Centre (DSDC) (2008) *Best Practice in Design for People with Dementia.* Stirling: University of Stirling.

Department of Constitutional Affairs (2007) *Mental Capacity Act 2005 Code of Practice.* London: TSO.

Department of Health (2007) *The Mental Capacity Act Deprivation of Liberty Safeguards.* London: DOH.

Department of Health (2008) *National End of Life Care Strategy: Promoting High Quality Care for All Adults at the End of Life.* London: DH Publications.

Department of Health (2009) *Living Well with Dementia: A National Dementia Strategy.* London: DH Publications.

Department of Health (2012) *Prime Minister's Challenge on Dementia: Delivering Major Improvements in Dementia and Research by 2015.* London: DH Publications.

Dewing, J. (2003) 'Rehabilitation for older people with dementia.' *Nursing Standard 18,* 6, 42–48.

Digby, R. and Bloomer, M.J. (2014) 'People with dementia and the hospital environment: the view of the patients and family carers.' *International Journal of Older People Nursing 9,* 1, 34–43.

Epp, T. (2003) 'Person-centred dementia care: a vision to be refined.' *Canadian Alzheimer Disease Review, April 2003,* 14–18.

Evans, D. (2002) 'A review of physical restraint minimization in the acute and residential care settings.' *Journal of Advanced Nursing 40,* 6, 616–625.

Evans, D., Wood, J. and Lambert, L. (2003) 'Patient injury and physical restraint devices. A systematic review.' *Journal of Advanced Nursing 41*, 3, 274–282.

Evans, G., Smith, A. and Morrow, K. (2009) *Compromised Swallowing: A Practical Guide to Nutrition, Hydration and Medication in Advanced Dementia.* Peterborough: Peterborough Palliative Care in Dementia Group. Accessed on 28/07/2016 at www.rcpsych.ac.uk/pdf/Dementia%20Compromised_swallowing_guide_July_2010.pdf

Eychmuller, S., Constantini, M. and Domeisen, F. (2012) 'OPCARE9 Work Package 1 – Signs and symptoms of approaching death.' *European Journal of Palliative Care 19*, 1, 20–23.

Family Caregiver Alliance (USA) (2013) *Grief and Loss.* San Francisco, CA: Family Caregiver Alliance. Accessed on 20/05/2016 at www.caregiver.org/grief-and-loss

Feil, N. (2002) *The Validation Breakthrough.* Baltimore, MD: Health Professions Press.

Gallinagh, R. (2002) 'The use of physical restraints as a safety measure in the care of older people in four rehabilitation wards. Findings from an exploratory study.' *International Journal of Nursing Studies 39*, 2, 147–156.

Gallinagh, R., Nevin, R., McAleese, L. and Campbell, L. (2001) 'Perceptions of older people who have experienced physical restraint.' *British Journal of Nursing 10*, 13, 852–859.

Gerrard, N. and Jones, J. (2016) *Voices from John's Campaign.* Chelmsford: Golden Duck.

Goldschmidt, B. and van Meines, N. (2011) *Comforting Touch in Dementia and End of Life Care.* London: Singing Dragon.

Granger, K. (2013) 'Hello my name is.' Accessed on 24/02/2016 at http://hellomynameis.org.uk

Guerchet, M., Prina, M., Prince, M., Albanese, E., Siervo, M. and Acosta, D. (2014) *Nutrition and Dementia.* London: Alzheimer's Disease International. Accessed on 19/04/2016 at www.alz.co.uk/sites/default/files/pdfs/nutrition-and-dementia.pdf

Gustafsson, C. and Fagerberg, I. (2004) 'Reflection, the way to professional development?' *Journal of Clinical Nursing 13*, 3, 271–280.

Hannan, R., Thompson, R., Worthington, A. and Rooney, P. (2015) *The Triangle of Care – Carers Included: A Guide to Best Practice for Dementia Care in Scotland.* Glasgow: Carers Trust. Accessed on 21/07/2016 at https://carers.org/sites/files/carerstrust/media/toc_scotland_dementia_final_0.pdf

Hannan, R., Thompson, R., Worthington, A. and Rooney, P. (2015) *The Triangle of Care – Carers Included: A Guide to Best Practice for Dementia Care.* London: Carers Trust. Accessed on 02/06/2016 at https://professionals.carers.org/sites/default/files/the_triangle_of_care_carers_included_best_practice_in_dementia_care_-_final.pdf

HarperCollins (1992) *Collins Softback English Dictionary.* Glasgow: HarperCollins.

Harrison Dening, K., King, M., Jones, L., Vickerstaff, V. and Sampson, E. (2016) 'Advanced care planning in dementia: do family carers know the treatment preferences of people with early dementia?' *PLOS ONE 11*, 7.

Health Innovation Network South London (2016) *What is Person-Centred Care and Why is it Important?* London: Health Innovation Network. Accessed on 09/08/2016 at www.hin-southlondon.org/system/ckeditor_assets/attachments/41/what_is_person-centred_care_and_why_is_it_important.pdf

Healthcare Improvement Scotland (2014) *Improving the Care for Older People – Delirium Toolkit.* Edinburgh: Healthcare Improvement Scotland. Accessed on 14/06/2016 at www.healthcareimprovementscotland.org/our_work/person-centred_care/opac_improvement_programme/delirium_toolkit.aspx

Henry, C. and Seymour, J. (2008) *Advance Care Planning: A Guide for Health and Social Care Staff.* Nottingham: University of Nottingham. Accessed on 13/06/2016 at www.ncpc.org.uk/sites/default/files/AdvanceCarePlanning.pdf

HM Government (2014) *Valuing every voice, respecting every right: Making the case for the Mental Capacity Act. The Government's response to the House of Lords Select Committee Report on the Mental Capacity Act 2005.* Policy Paper. London: HMSO.

Hughes, R. (ed.) (2010) *Rights, Risks and Restraint-Free Care for Older People.* London: Jessica Kingsley Publishers.

Husebo, B., Ballard, C., Sandvik, R., Bjarte Nilsen, O. and Aarsland, D. (2011) 'Efficacy of treating pain to reduce behavioural disturbances in residents of nursing homes with dementia: cluster randomised clinical trial.' *British Medical Journal 343*, d4065.

Institute of Neuroscience, Trinity College Dublin (2014) *Hello Brain Project.* Dublin: Trinity College Dublin. Accessed on 28/06/2016 at www.hellobrain.eu/en

Institute of Neuroscience, Trinity College Dublin (2015) *Hello Brain Project.* Dublin: Trinity College Dublin. Accessed on 20/06/2016 at www.hellobrain.eu/en

James, I. (2011) *Understanding Behavioural in Dementia that Challenges: A Guide to Assessment and Treatment.* London: Jessica Kingsley Publishers.

John's Campaign (2016) *Resources.* London: John's Campaign. Accessed on 18/08/2016 at www.johnscampaign.org.uk/resources

Jootun, D. and Pryde, A. (2013) 'Moving and handling of patients with dementia.' *Journal of Nursing Education and Practice 3*, 2, 127.

Judd, S., Marshall, M. and Phippen, P. (1998) *Design For Dementia.* London: Hawker Publications.

Keltner, D. (2010) *Hands On Research: The Science of Touch.* Berkeley, CA: University of California. Accessed on 27/05/2016 at http://greatergood.berkeley.edu/article/item/hands_on_research

Kendall, K. (2015) *Everything You Need to Know About Hydration.* Boise, ID: Bodybuilding.com. Accessed on 31/08/2016 at www.bodybuilding. com/fun/everything-you-need-to-know-about-hydration. html?mcid=infographic

Killick, J. and Allan, K. (2001) *Communication and the Care of People with Dementia.* Buckingham: Open University Press.

Kitwood, T. (1997) *Dementia Reconsidered: The Person Comes First.* New York, NY: Open University Press.

Lakey, L. (Alzheimer's Society) (2009) *Counting the Cost: Caring for People with Dementia on Hospital Wards.* London: Alzheimer's Society. Accessed on 22/07/2016 at www.alzheimers.org.uk/site/scripts/download_info. php?fileID=787

Lighting for Health (2013) *What is Biodynamic Light?* Manchester: Lighting for Health. Accessed on 20/08/2016 at http://lightingforhealth.com/biodynamic-lighting-2

Lord, K., White, N., Scott, S. and Sampson, E.L. (2013) 'The Behaviour and Pain (Bepaid) Study: dementia patients who die in the acute hospital.' *British Medical Journal, Supportive Palliative Care 3*, 1, 24–125.

MacNeill, S.A. and Licthenberg, P.A. (1997) 'Home alone: the role of cognition in return to independent living.' *Physical Medicine and Rehabilitation 78*, 7, 755–758.

McCloskey, R. (2004) 'Caring for patients with dementia in an acute care environment.' *Geriatric Nursing 25*, 3, 139–144.

McKeefry, D. and Bartlett, R. (2010) *Improving Vision and Eye Health Care to People with Dementia.* London: Thomas Pocklington Trust. Accessed on 02/05/2016 at http://pocklington-trust.org.uk/wp-content/uploads/2016/02/RDP8.pdf

McLean, W. and Cunningham, C. (2007) *Pain in Older People and People with Dementia: A Practical Guide.* Stirling: The Dementia Services Development Centre, Stirling University Press.

May, H., Edwards, E. and Brooker, D. (2009) *Enriched Care Planning for People with Dementia.* London: Jessica Kingsley Publishers.

Melzack, R. and Casey, K.L. (1968) 'Sensory, Motivational and Central Control Determinants of Chronic Pain: A New Conceptual Model.' In D.R. Kenshalo (ed.) *The Skin Senses: Proceedings of the First International Symposium on the Skin Senses, Held at the Florida State University in Tallahassee.* Springfield, IL: Charles C. Thomas.

Mental Capacity Act (2005) London: HMSO.

Menzies, I.B., Mendelson, D.A., Kates, S.L. and Friedman, S.M. (2010) 'Prevention and clinical management of hip fractures in patients with dementia.' *Geriatric Orthopaedic Surgery & Rehabilitation 1*, 2, 63–72.

Ministry of Justice (2008) *Mental Capacity Act 2005: Deprivation of Liberty Safeguards – Code of Practice to supplement the main Mental Capacity Act 2005 Code of Practice.* Supplement paper. London: TSO.

Morrison, R.S. and Siu, A.L. (2000) 'A comparison of pain and its treatment in advanced dementia and cognitively impaired patients with hip fracture.' *Journal of Pain Symptom Management 19*, 4, 240–248.

National End of Life Team (2008) *Advance Care Planning: A Guide for Health and Social Care Staff*. NHS England. Accessed on 13/06/2016 at www.ncpc. org.uk/sites/default/files/AdvanceCarePlanning.pdf

National Institute for Clinical Excellence (NICE) and Social Care Institute for Excellence (SCIE) (2006) *Dementia – Supporting People with Dementia and their Carers in Health and Social Care*. Leicester: The British Psychological Society and Gaskell. Accessed on 09/08/16 at www.nice.org.uk/guidance/cg42/ chapter/introduction

National Institute for Health and Clinical Excellence (NICE) (2010) *Delirium: Prevention, Diagnosis and Management*. Manchester: NICE. Accessed on 31/04/2016 at www.nice.org.uk/guidance/cg103/resources/ delirium-prevention-diagnosis-and-management-35109327290821

National Patient Safety Agency (NPSA) (2005) *Bedrails – Reviewing the Evidence. A Systematic Literature Review*. London: NPSA. Accessed on 10/03/2016 at www.nrls.npsa.nhs.uk/EasySiteWeb/getresource.axd?AssetID=61400

Newbronner, L., Chamberlain, R., Borthwick, R., Baxter, M. and Glendinning, C. (2013) *A Road Less Rocky*. London: Carer's Trust. Accessed on 15/08/2016 at https://carers.org/sites/files/carerstrust/media/ dementia_executive_summary_english_only_final_use_this_one.pdf

NHS Choices (2015) *Your Care After Discharge from Hospital*. London: NHS. Accessed on 25/07/2016 at www.nhs.uk/conditions/social-care-and-support-guide/pages/hospital-discharge-care.aspx

NHS Emergency Care Intensive Support Team (NHS ECIST) (2012) *Whole System Priorities for the Discharge of Frail Older People from Hospital Care*. London: NHS ECIST. Accessed on 03/05/2016 at www.england.nhs.uk/ wp-content/uploads/2013/08/dis-old-people.pdf

NHS England (2016) *Commissioning for Quality and Innovation (CQUIN) Guidance for 2016/2017*. London: NHS England. Accessed on 17/08/2016 at www. england.nhs.uk/wp-content/uploads/2016/03/cquin-guidance-16-17-v3.pdf

NHS Interim Management and Support (NHS IMAS) (2012) *Effective Approaches in Urgent and Emergency Care – Paper 3 – Whole System Priorities for the Discharge of Frail Older People from Hospital Care*. London: NHS IMAS. Accessed on 08/04/2016 at www.nhsimas.nhs.uk/fileadmin/Files/ ECIST_Conference_October_2012/ECIST_papers/FINAL_ECIST_ Paper_3_-__Priorities_for_Discharging_Older_People_from_Hospital_1_ October_2012.pdf

Parker, G. (2014) *Intermediate Care, Reablement or Something Else? A Research Note about the Challenges of Defining Services*. York: University of York. Accessed on 15/08/2016 at www.york.ac.uk/inst/spru/pubs/pdf/ICR.pdf

Parkinson's UK (2016) *Get It on Time*. London: Parkinson's UK. Accessed on 11/08/2016 at www.parkinsons.org.uk/content/get-it-time

Partridge, R. and Campbell, C. (2007) *Artificial Nutrition and Hydration Guidance in End of Life Care for Adults.* London: National Council for Palliative Care and the Association of Palliative Medicine.

Philp, I. (2007) *Foreword: The Assessment of Pain in Older People: National Guidelines.* London: Royal College of Physicians, British Geriatrics Society and British Pain Society. Accessed on 12/07/2016 at www.britishpainsociety.org/static/uploads/resources/files/book_pain_older_people.pdf

Power, G.A. (2014) *Dementia Beyond Disease: Enhancing Well-being.* Baltimore: Health Professions Press.

Power, A.G. (2015) 'Well-being: a strength based approach to dementia.' *Australian Journal of Dementia Care.* Accessed on 11/06/2016 at www.journalofdementiacare.com/well-being-a-strengths-based-approach-to-dementia

Remington, R., Abdullah, L., Melillo, K. and Flanagan, J. (2006) 'Managing problem behaviours associated with dementia.' *Rehabilitation Nursing 31,* 5, 186–192.

Ronch, J.L., Bradley, A.M., Pohlmann, E., Cummings, N.A. *et al.* (2004) 'The Electronic Dementia Guide for Excellence (EDGE): an internet education programme for care of residents with dementia in nursing homes.' *Alzheimer's Care Quarterly 5,* 3, 230–240.

Rösler, A., Pfeil, S., Lessmann, H., Höder, J., Befahr, A. and von Renteln-Kruse, W. (2015) 'Dysphagia in dementia: influence of dementia severity and food texture on the prevalence of aspiration and latency to swallow in hospitalized geriatric patients.' *Journal of American Medical Director's Association 16,* 8, 697–701.

Royal College of Nursing (RCN) (2008) *Let's Talk About Restraints: Rights, Risks and Responsibility.* London: RCN.

Royal National Institute of Blind People (RNIB) and Alzheimer's Scotland (2012) *Dementia and Sight Loss.* London: RNIB and Alzheimer Scotland. Accessed on 19/07/2016 at www.rnib.org.uk/sites/default/files/Dementia_and_sight_loss_leaflet.pdf

Sampson, E.L., Candy, B. and Jones, L. (2009) 'Enteral tube feeding for older people with advanced dementia.' *The Cochrane Database of Systematic Reviews 2,* 4.

Sander, R. (2002) 'Standing and moving: helping people with vascular dementia.' *Nursing Older People 14,* 1, 20–26.

Social Care Institute for Excellence (SCIE) (2015) *End of Life Care and Carers' Needs.* London: Social Care Institute for Excellence. Accessed on 18/05/2016 at www.scie.org.uk/dementia/advanced-dementia-and-end-of-life-care/end-of-life-care/carers-needs.asp

Shepherd, G., Boardman, J. and Slade, M. (2008) *Making Recovery a Reality.* London: Sainsbury Centre for Mental Health.

Sinclair, A. and Dickinson, E. (1998) *Effective Practice in Rehabilitation: The Evidence of Systematic Reviews.* London: King's Fund.

Stokes, G. (2010) *And Still the Music Plays.* London: Hawker Publications.

Taylor, R. (2015) *Alzheimer's From the Inside Out.* Baltimore, MD: Health Professions Press.

Thompson, F., Girling, D., Green, S. and Wai, C. (2010) 'Care of People with Dementia in the General Hospital.' In M. Downes and B. Bowers (eds) *Excellence in Dementia Care: Research into Practice.* Maidenhead: Open University Press.

Thompson, R. (2011) 'Using life story work to enhance care.' *Nursing Older People 23,* 8, 16–21.

Tresolini, C. (1994) *The Pew Fetzer Task Force on Psychosocial Education. Health Professions Education and Relationship-Centered Care: Report of the Pew-Fetzer Task Force on Advancing Psychosocial Education.* San Francisco, CA: Pew Health Professions Commission. Accessed on 18/06/2016 at www.rccswmi.org/uploads/PewFetzerRCCreport.pdf

Tritter, J. and Koivusalo, M. (2013) 'Undermining patient and public engagement and limiting its impact: the consequences of the Health and Social Care Act 2012 on collective patient and public involvement.' *Health Expectations: An International Journal of Public Participation in Health Care and Health Policy 16,* 2, 115–118.

Twycross, R. and Lack, S. (1983) *Symptom Control in Far Advanced Cancer: Pain Relief.* London: Pitman Books.

United Kingdom Supreme Court (2014) *P v Cheshire West and Chester Council* and *P and Q v Surrey County Council.* MHLO 16 (UKSC); 19

Van Hoof, J., Kort, H.S.M., Duijnstee, M.S.H., Rutten, P.G.S and Hensen, J.L.M. (2010) 'The indoor environment and the integrated design of homes for older people with dementia.' *Building and Environment 45,* 5, 1244–1261.

Varnam, W. (2011) 'How to mobilise patients with dementia to a standing position.' *Nursing Older People 23,* 8, 31–36.

Waite, J., Harwood, R.H., Morton, I.R. and Connelly, D.J. (2009) *Dementia Care: A Practical Manual.* New York, NY: Oxford University Press.

Warden, V., Hurley, A.C. and Volicer, L. (2003) 'Development and psychometric evaluation of the pain assessment in advanced dementia (PAINAD) scale.' *Journal of American Medical Directors Association 4,* 1, 9–15.

Woods, A.T., Poliakoff, E., Lloyd, D.M., Kuenzel, J. *et al.* (2011) 'Effect of background noise on food perception.' *Food Quality and Preference 22,* 1, 42–47.

World Health Organisation (WHO) (1948) *Definition of Health.* Geneva: WHO. Accessed on 22/06/2016 at www.who.int/about/definition/en/print.html

World Health Organisation (WHO) (1990) *Dementia.* Geneva: WHO. Accessed on 18/04/2016 at www.who.int/topics/dementia/en

World Health Organisation (WHO) (2015) *WHO Thematic Briefing: Ensuring a Human Rights-Based Approach for People Living with Dementia.* Geneva: WHO. Accessed on 29/03/2016 at www.ohchr.org/Documents/Issues/OlderPersons/Dementia/ThematicBrief.pdf

Wright, K. (2005) 'Mobility and safe handling of people with dementia.' *Nursing Times 101*, 17, 38–40.

Young, J. and Inouye, S. (2007) 'Delirium in older people.' *British Medical Journal 334*, 7598, 842–846.

Ziesel, J. (2010) *I'm Still Here – Creating a Better Life for a Loved One Living with Alzheimer's.* London: Little Brown Book Group.

Useful Websites

British Geriatrics Society – www.bgs.org.uk

British Pain Society – www.britishpainsociety.org

Healthcare Improvement Scotland – www.healthcareimprovementscotland.org

Mental Capacity Act 2005 Code of Practice – www.gov.uk/government/uploads/system/uploads/attachment_data/file/497253/Mental-capacity-act-code-of-practice.pdf

National Council for Palliative Care – www.ncpc.org.uk/publication/how-would-I-know

The Pain Centre – www.paincentrenapp.co.uk

Social Care Institute for Excellence – www.scie.org.uk

Subject Index

Author Index